SPOT THE DIFFERENCES

BOOK FOR SENIORS

AND ELDERLY WITH DEMENTIA, PARKINSON'S, AND ALZHEIMER'S

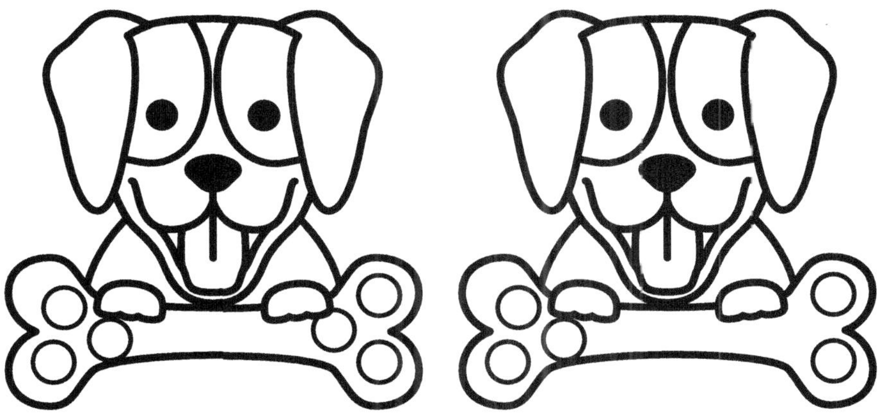

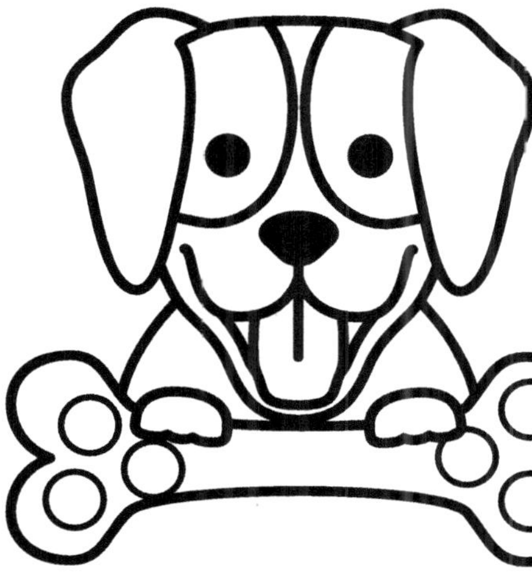

THIS BOOK BELONGS TO:

Welcome

This coloring book features EASY and FUN spot the difference activity pages for Seniors to enjoy!

We hope that you enjoy this book and would love for you to check out the other Activity Books and Coloring books that we have available in our collection. Enjoy!

Plush Prints Publishing

How it Works

The goal is to find the image that looks different from the other images on each page.

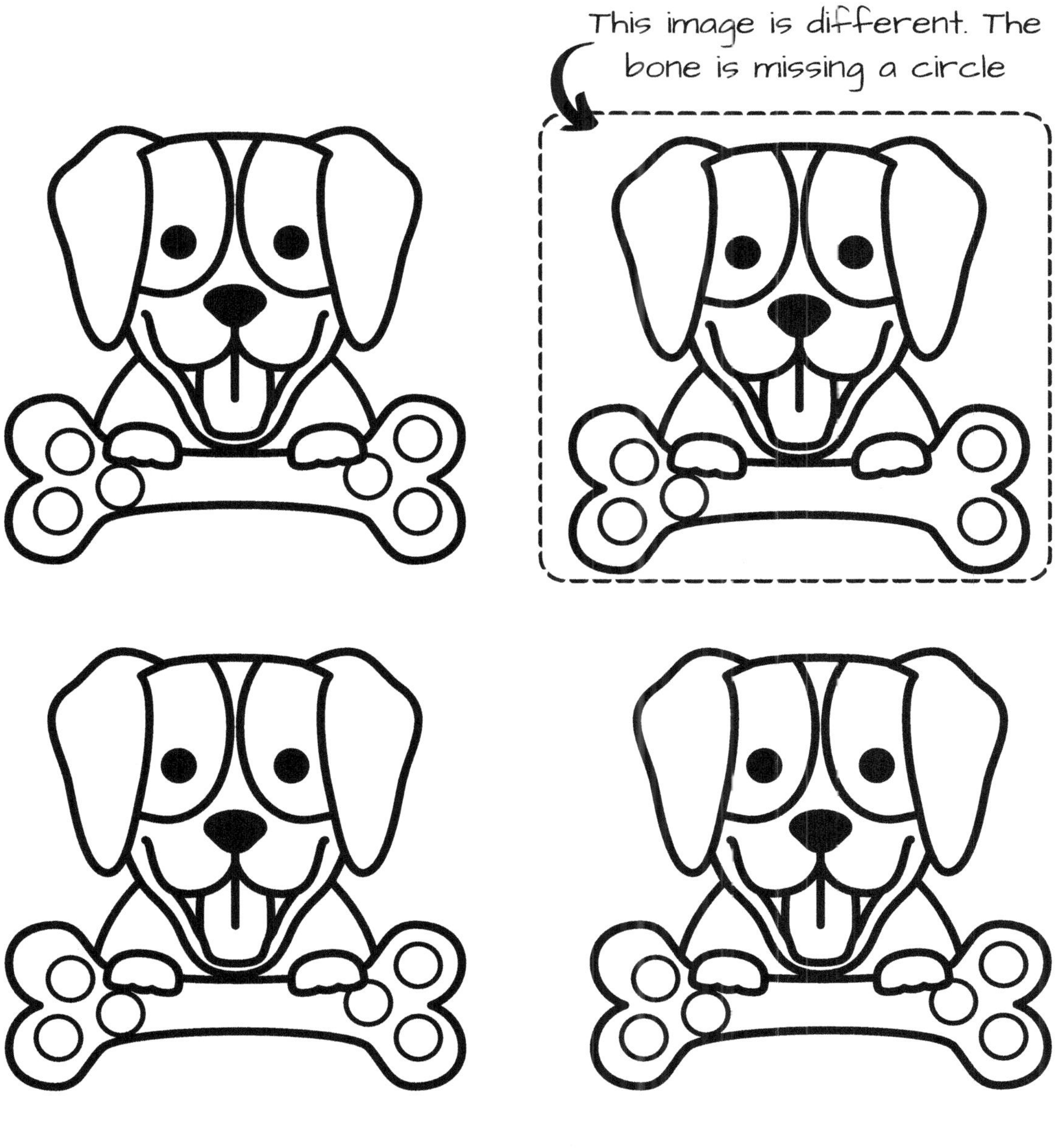

Find the Bird that is Different from the Others

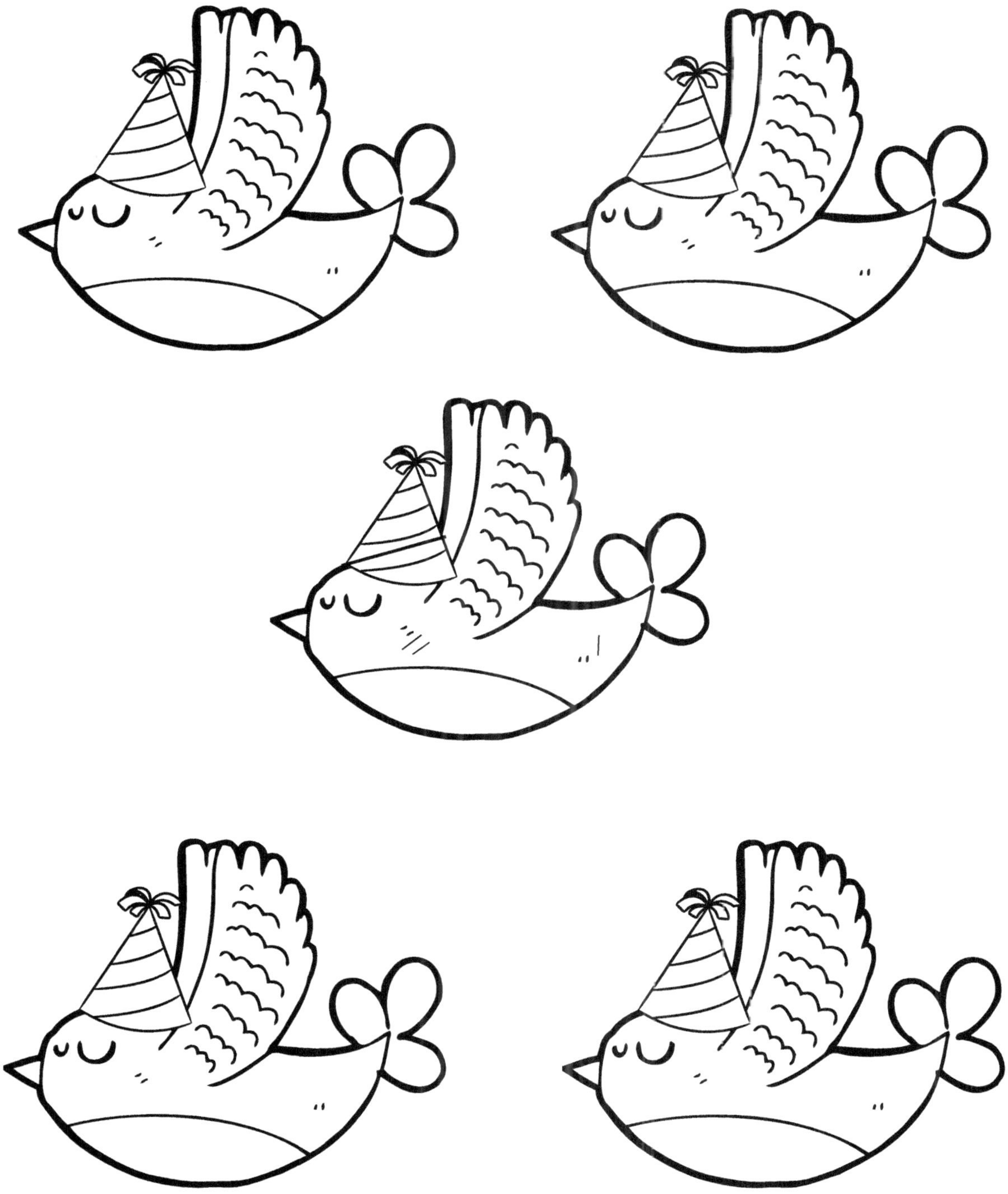

Find the Sand Pale that is Different from the Others

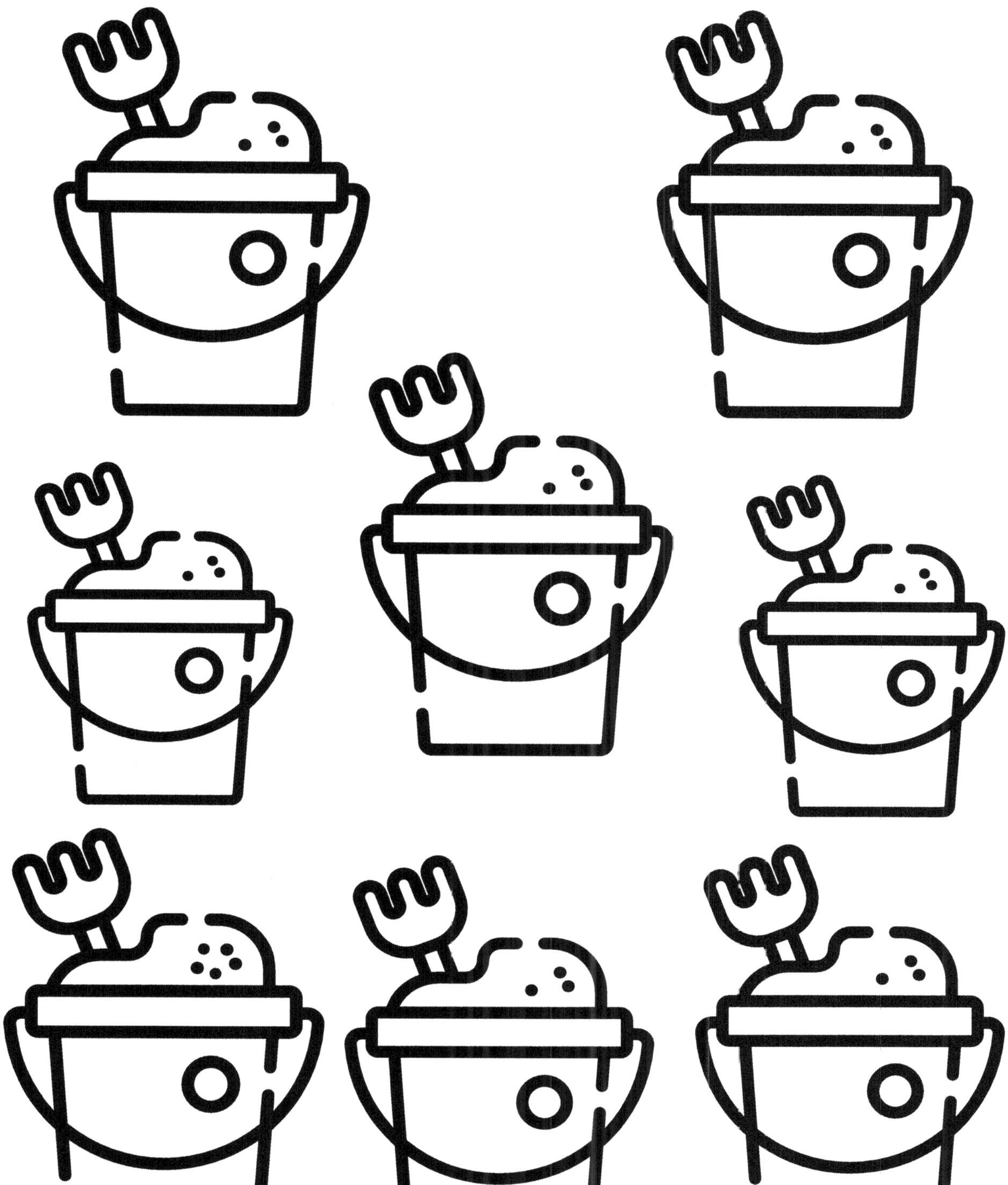

Find the Pair of Glasses that are Different from the Others

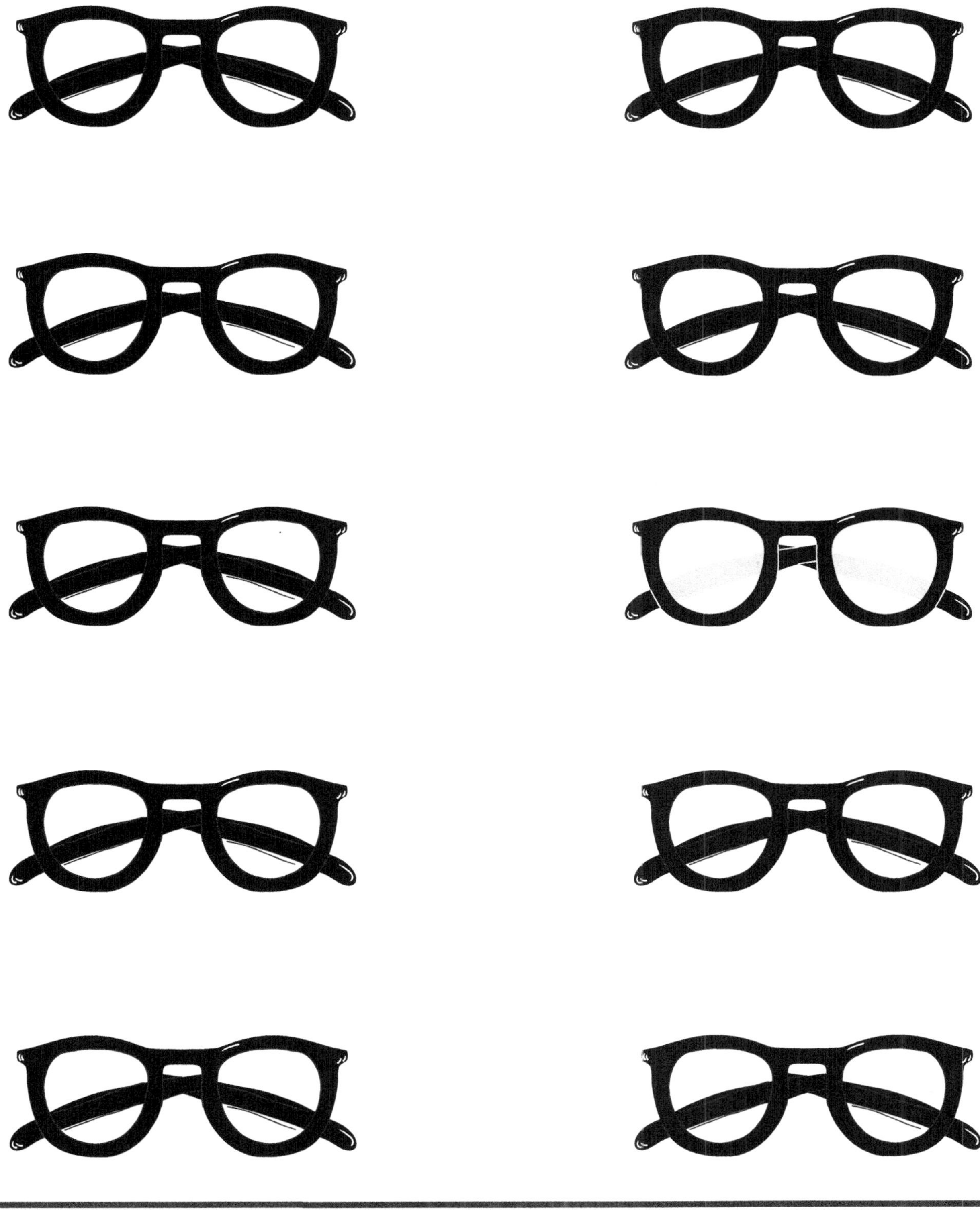

Find the Pair of shorts that are Different from the Others

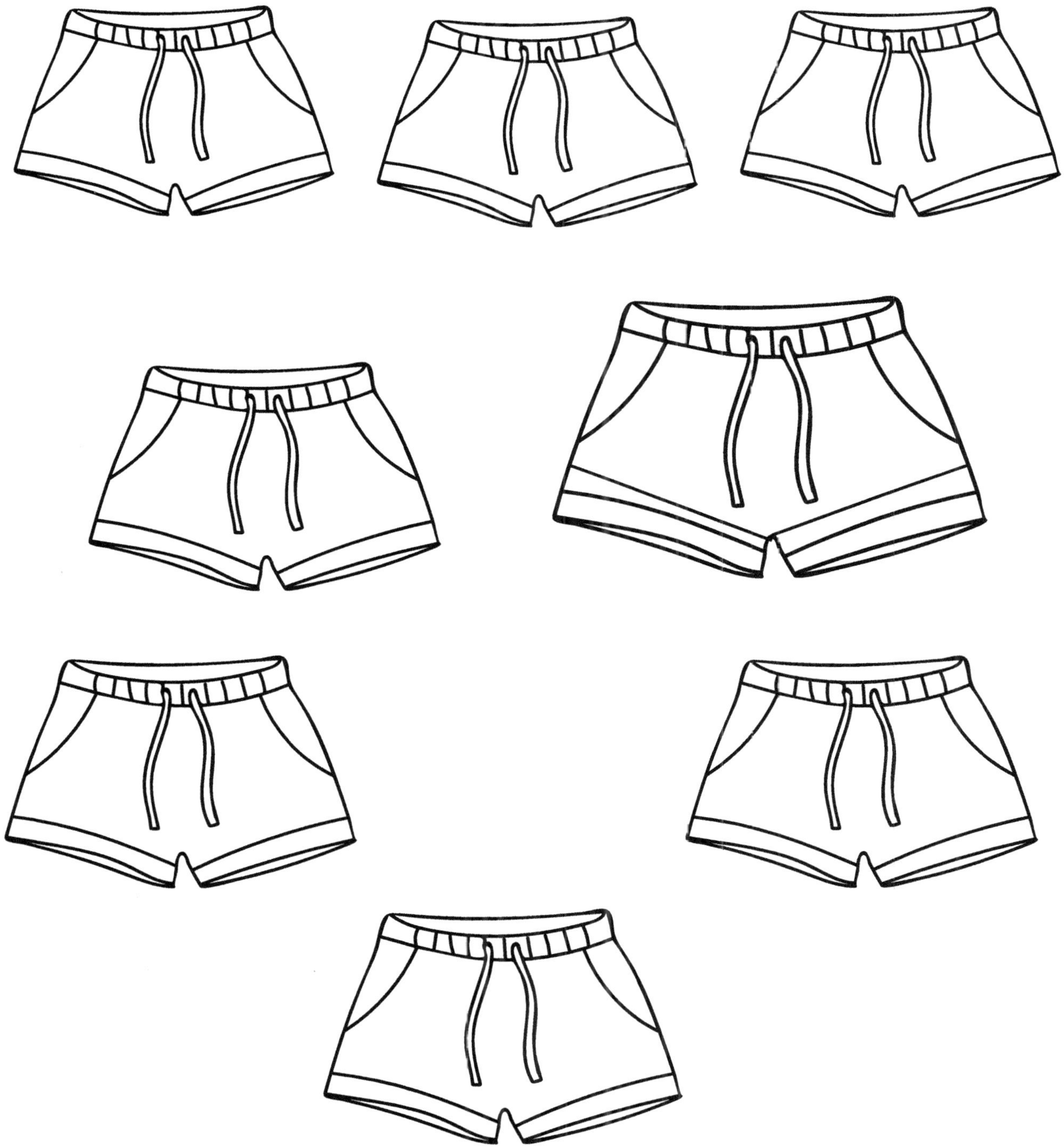

Find the plant that are Different from the Others

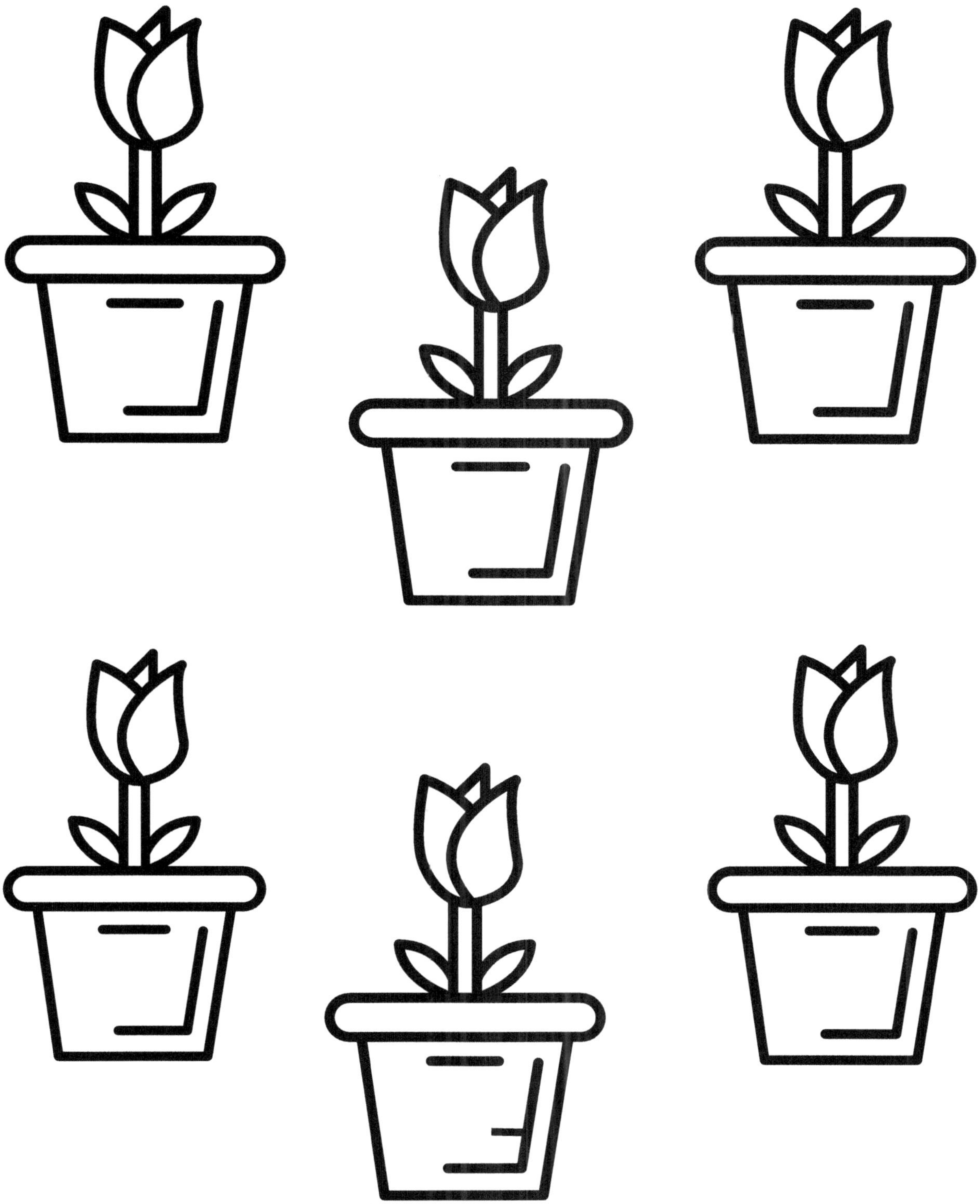

Find the wheelbarrow that are Different from the Others

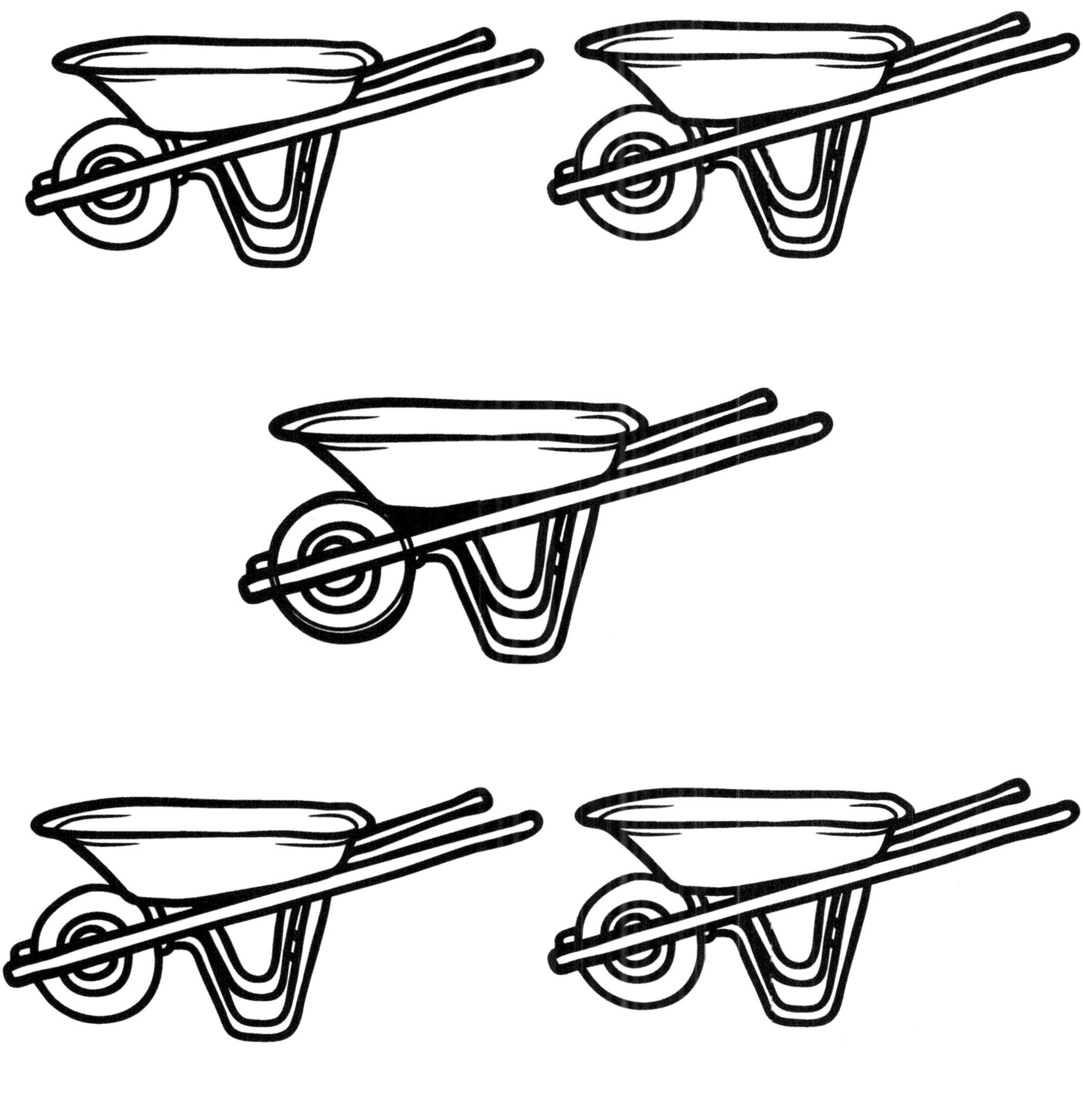

Find the Lamp that is Different from the Others

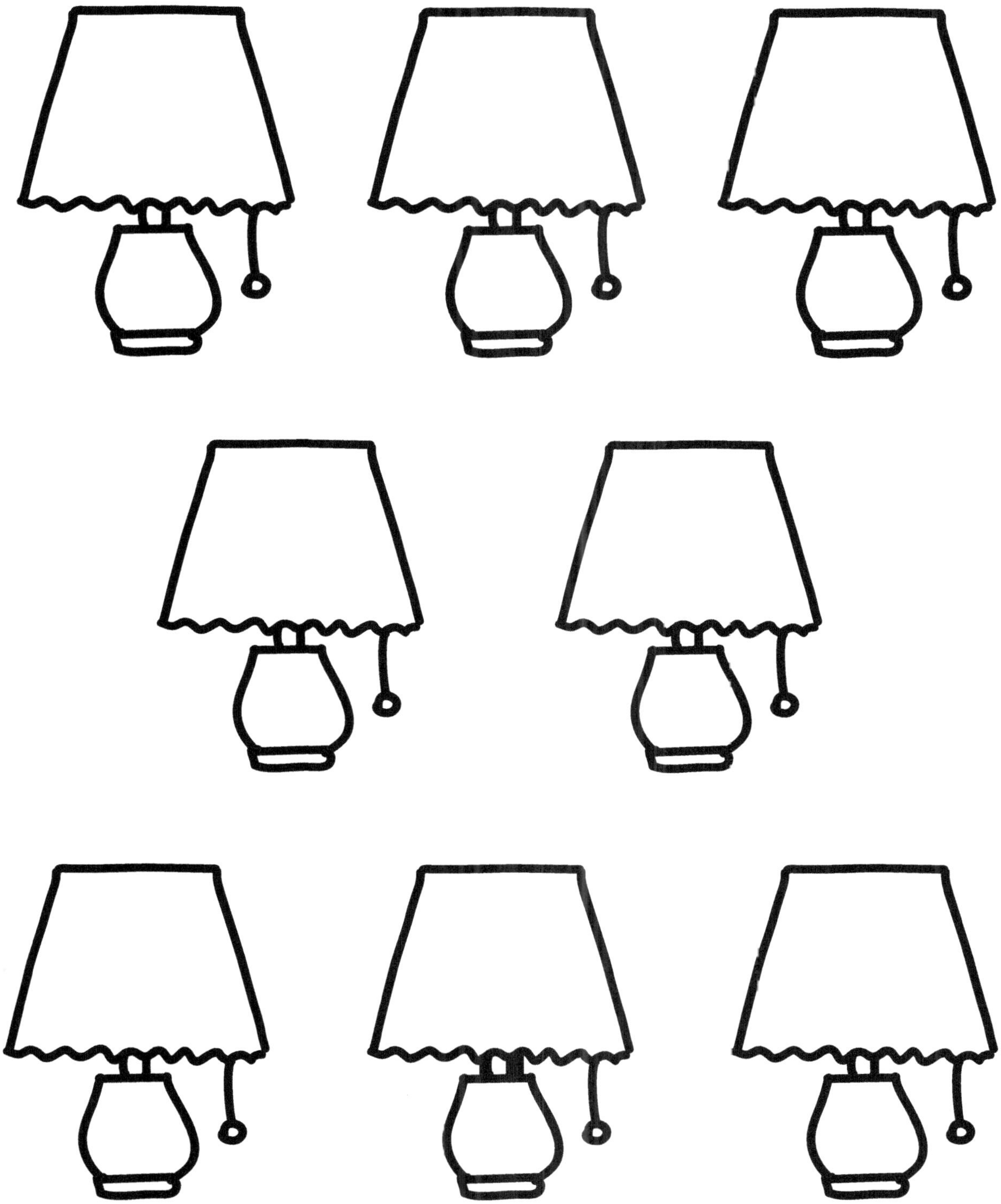

Find the Door that is Different from the Others

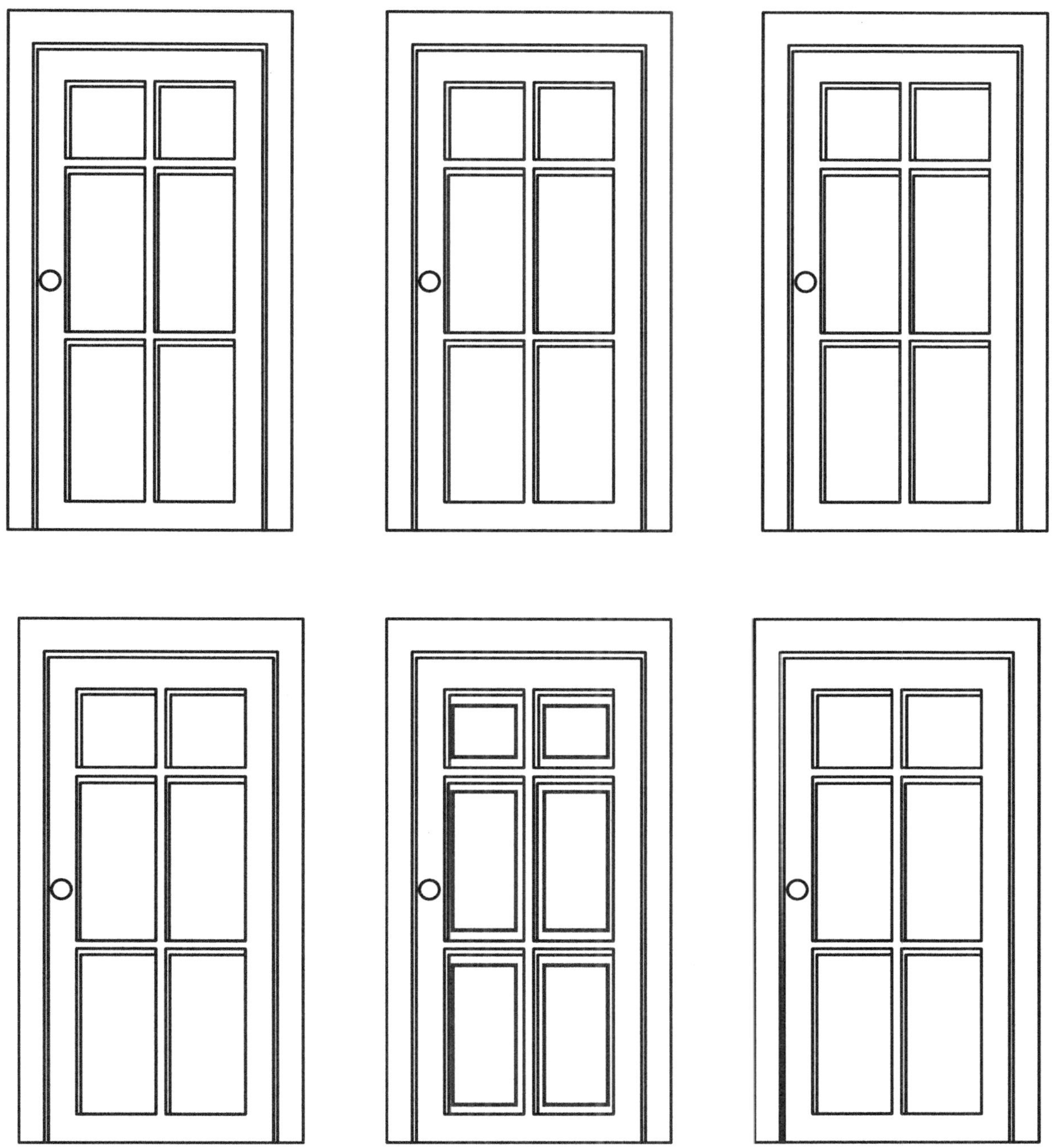

Find the Backpack that is Different from the Others

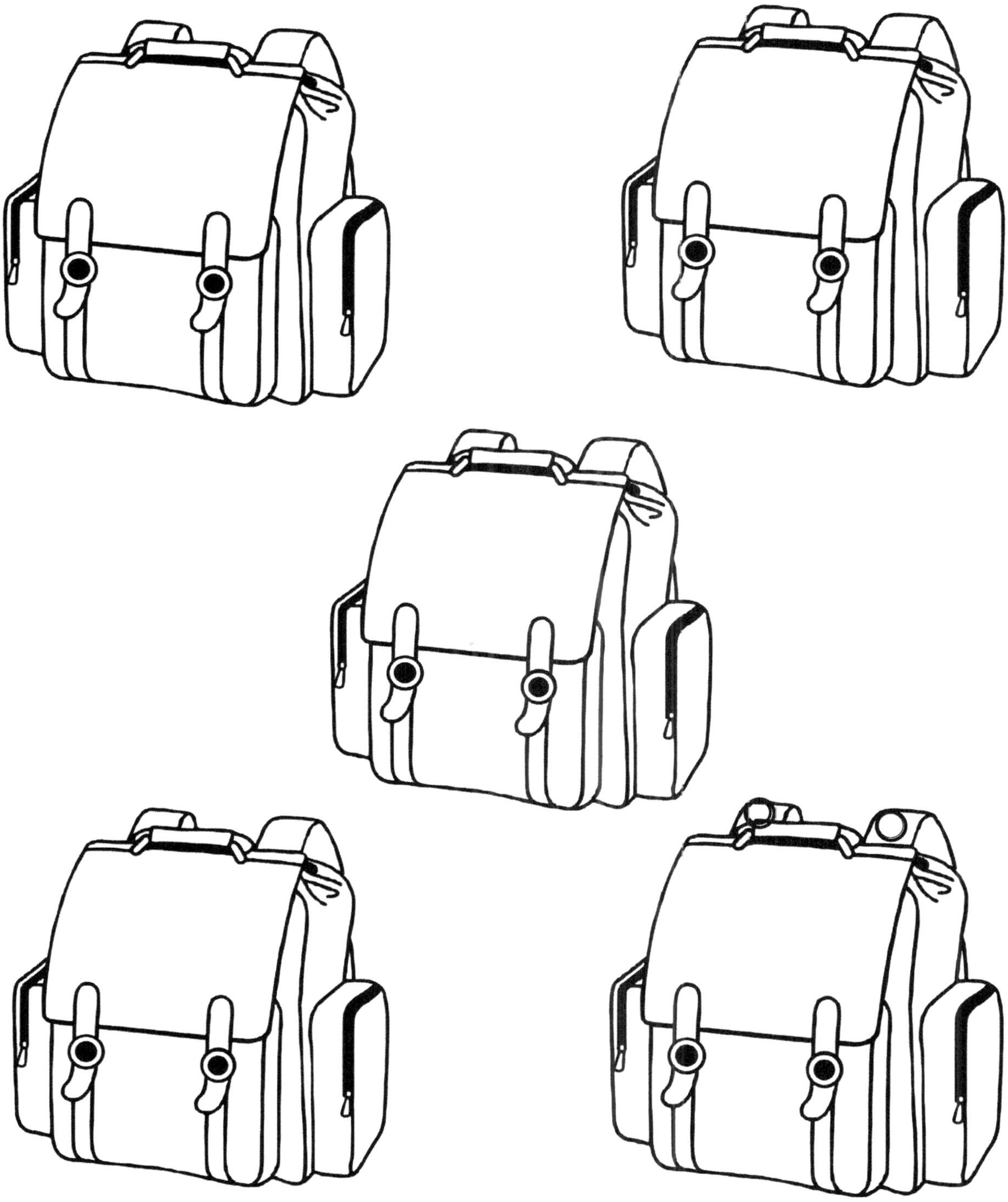

Find the Car that is Different from the Others

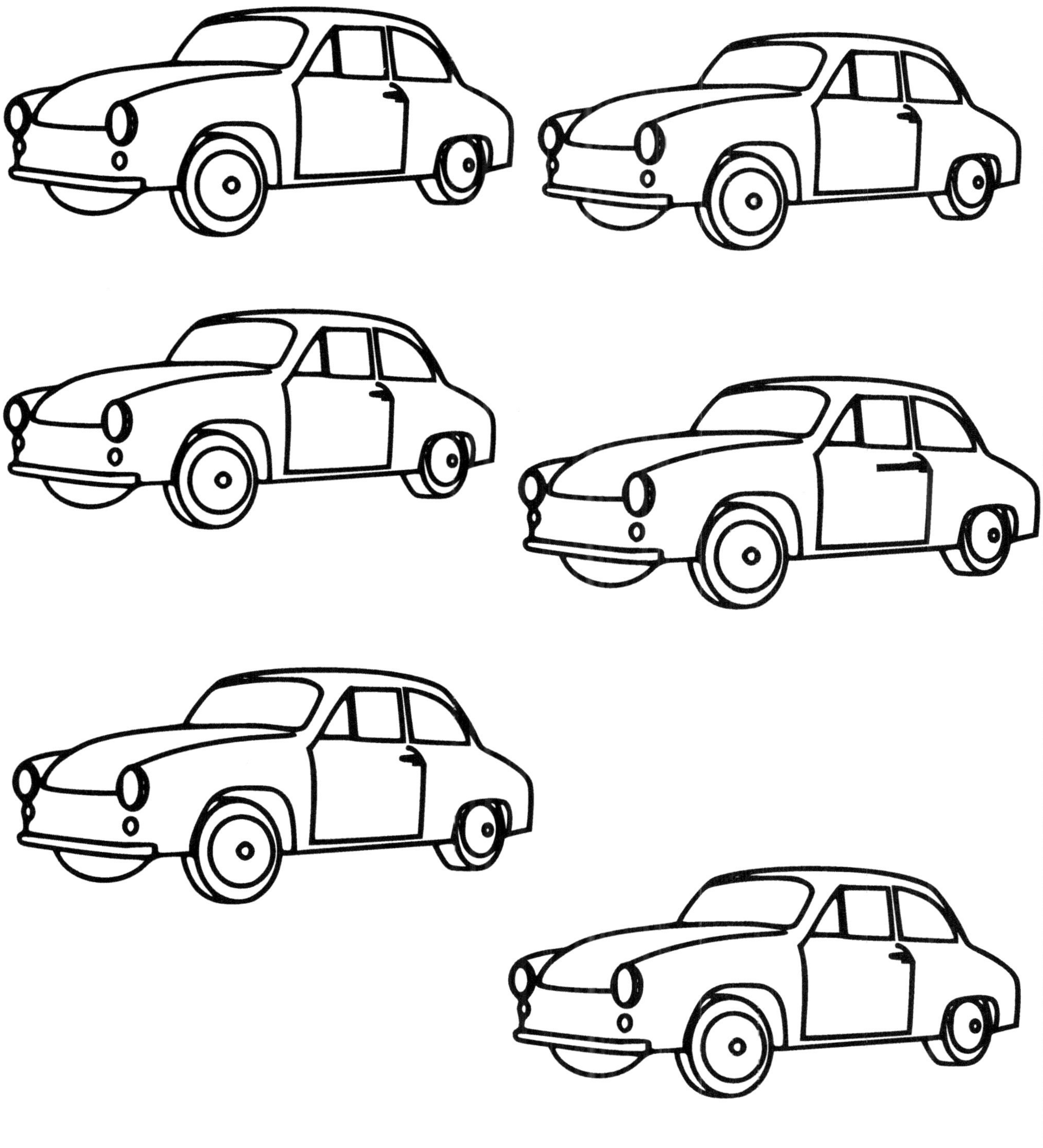

Find the Guitar that is Different from the Others

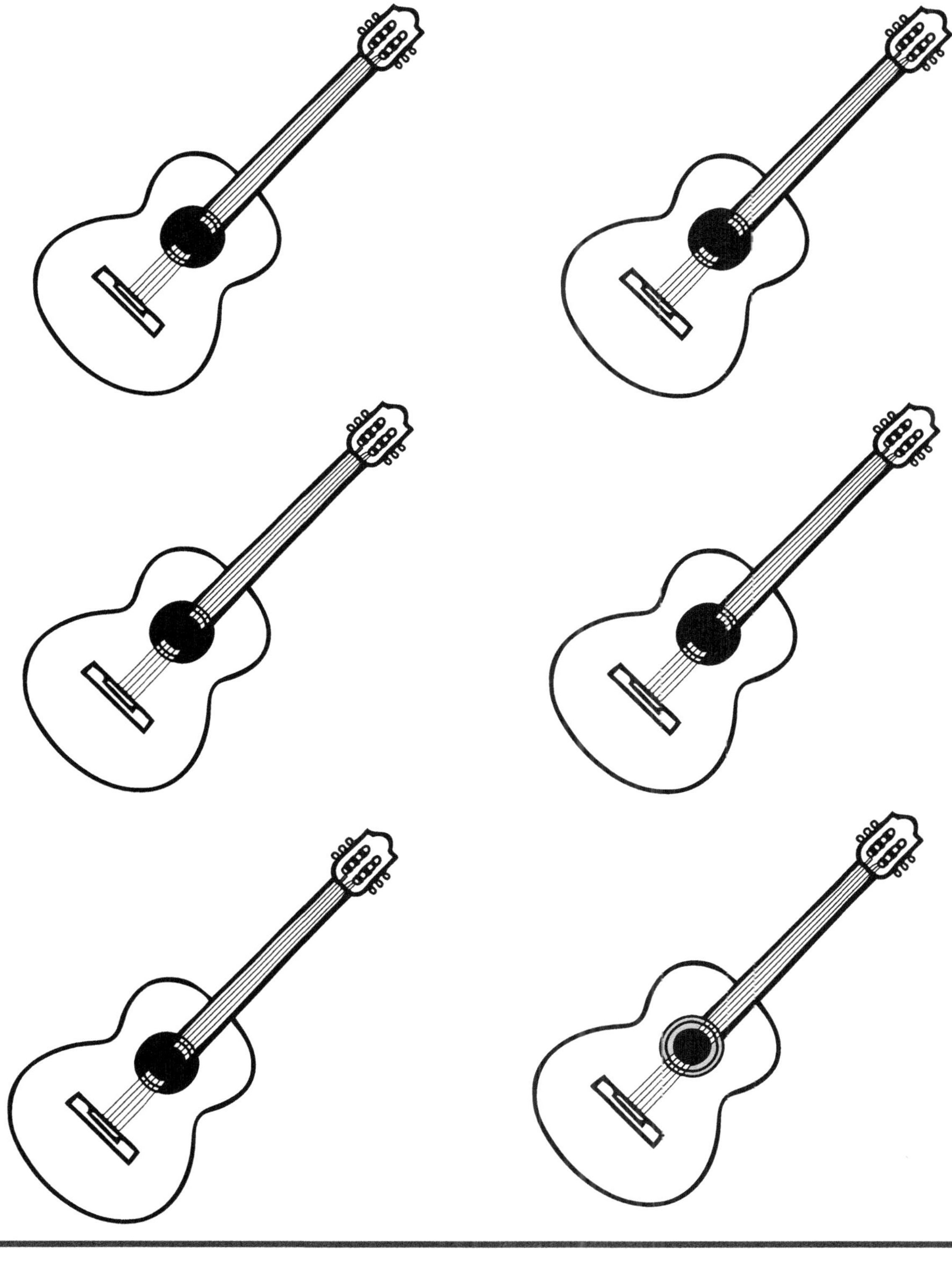

Find the House that is Different from the Others

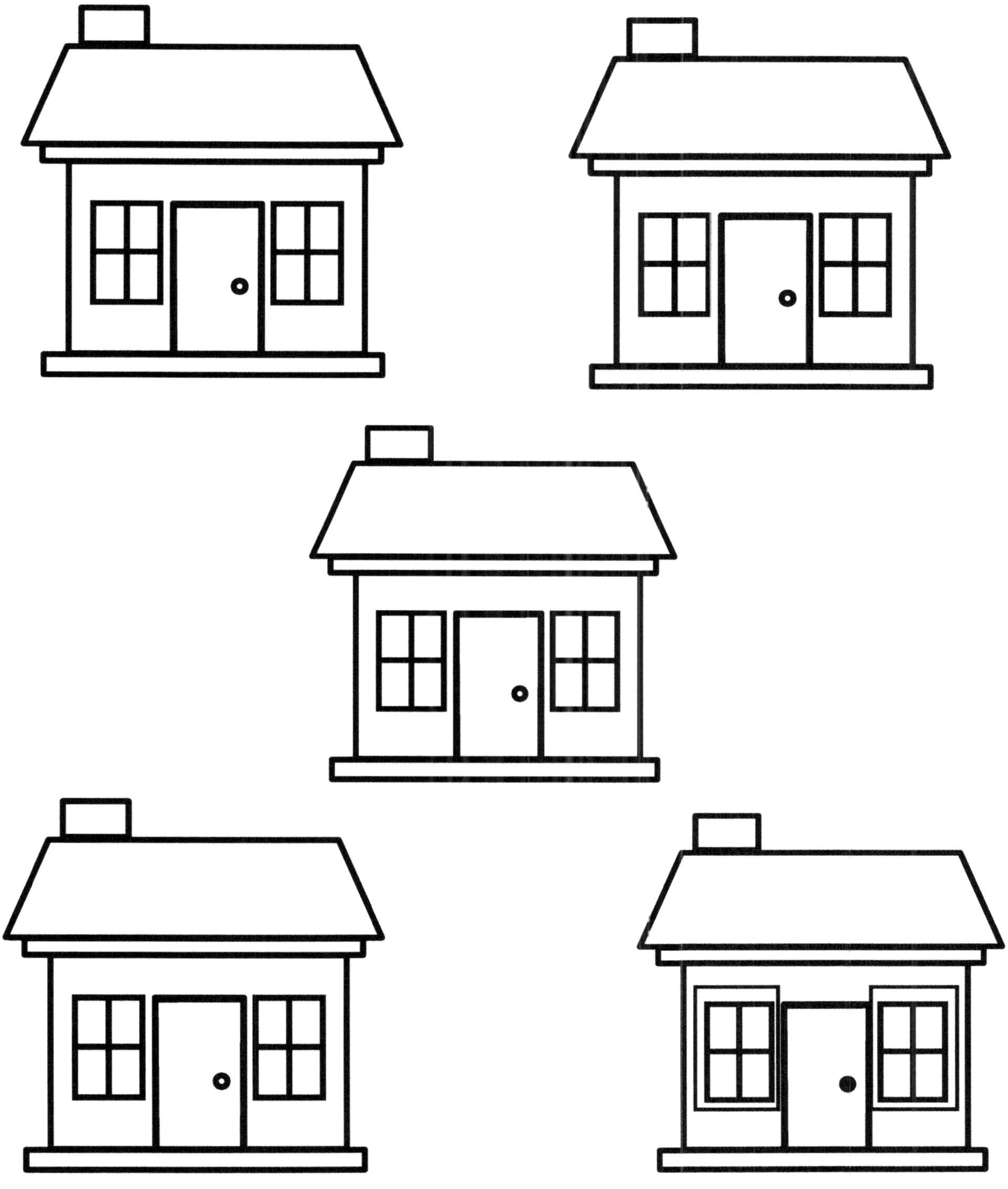

Find the Gardening picture that is Different from the Others

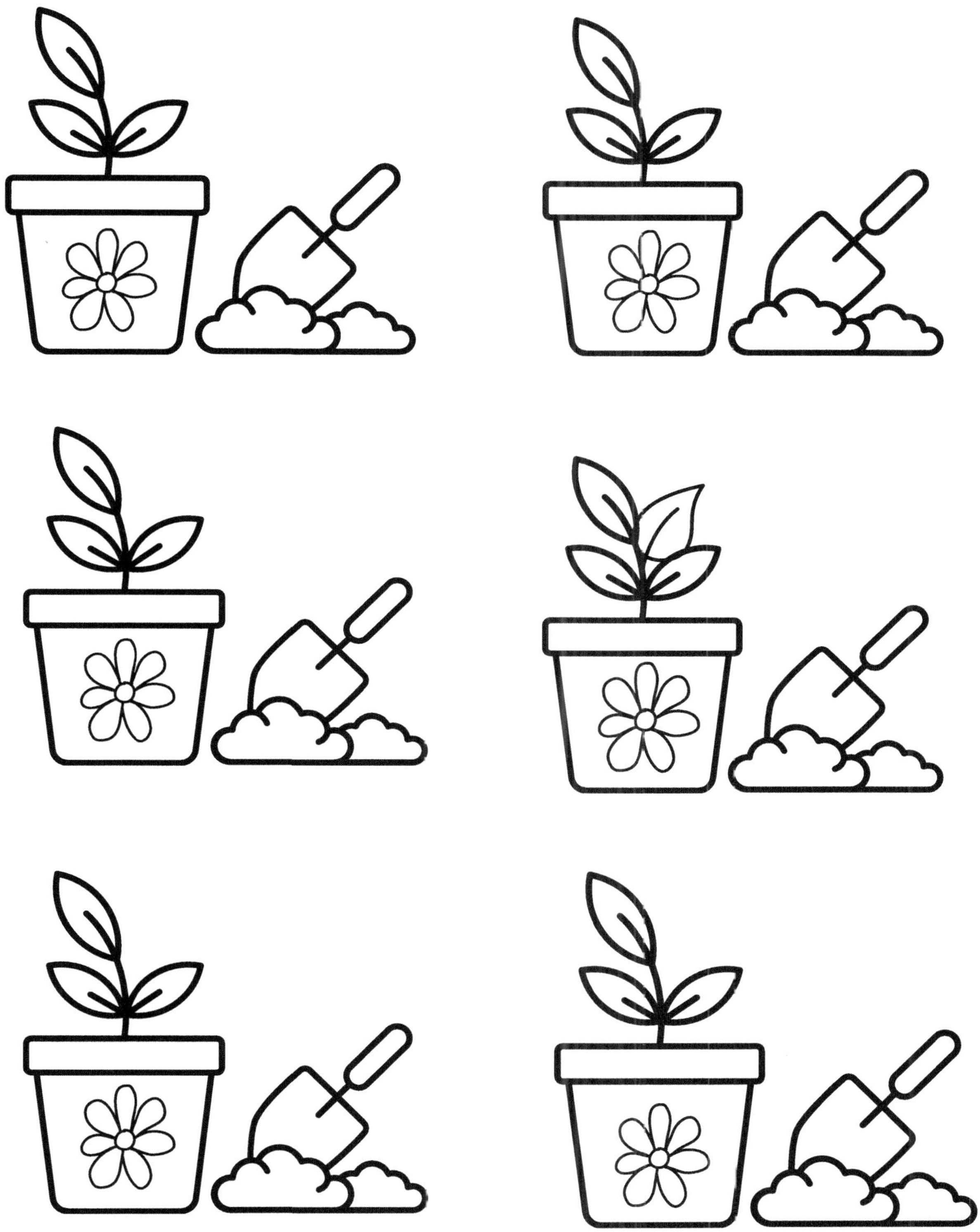

Find the Barn that is Different from the Others

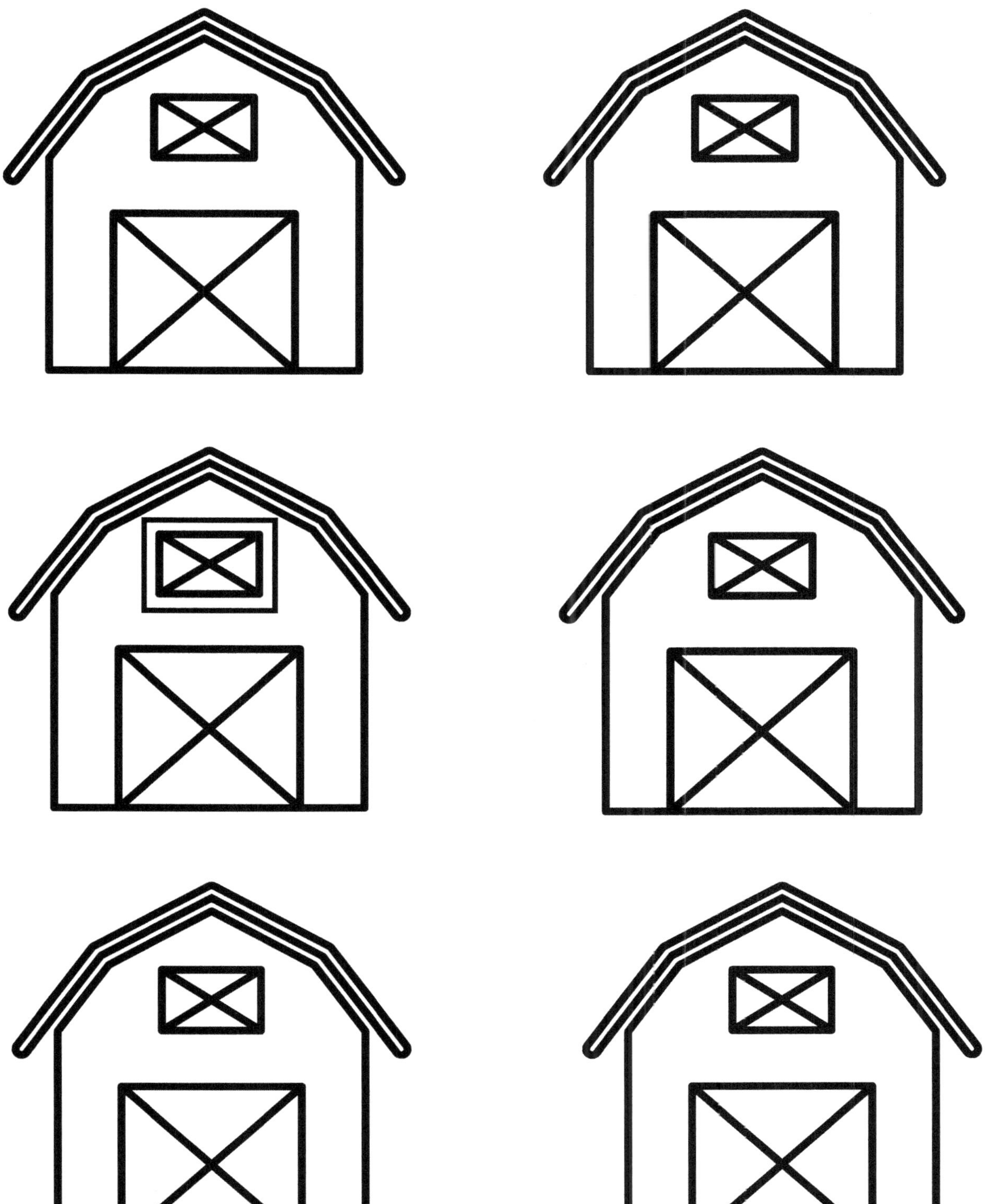

Find the Pinata that is Different from the Others

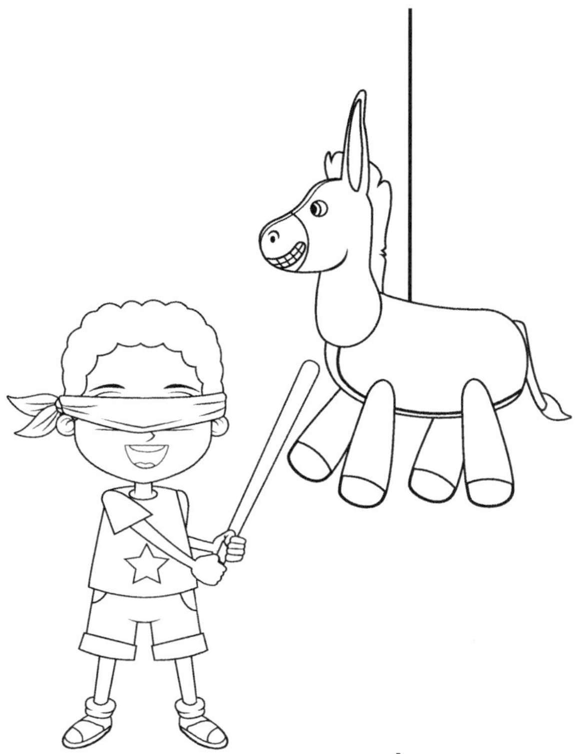

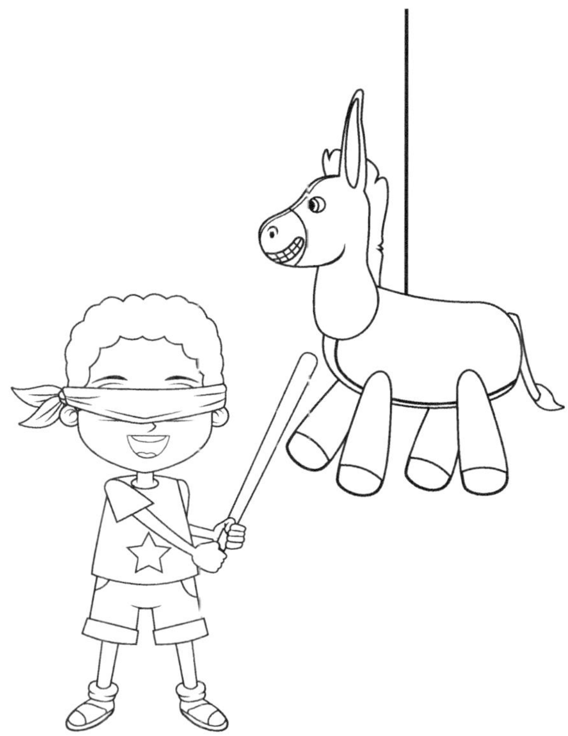

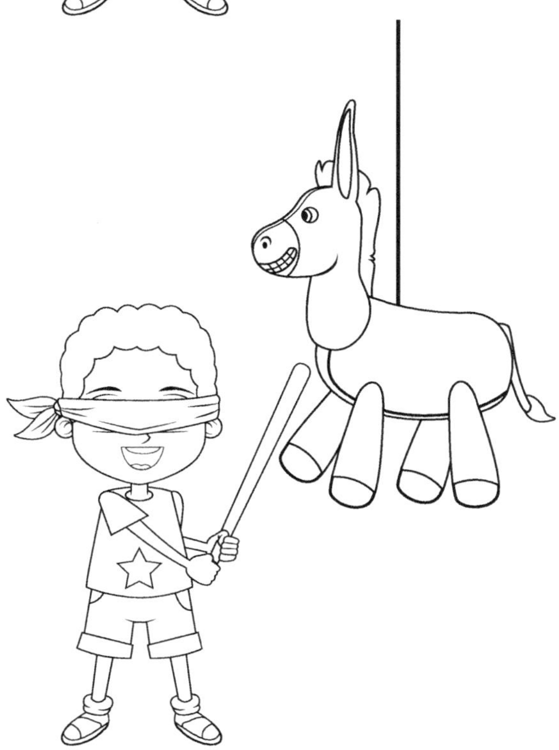

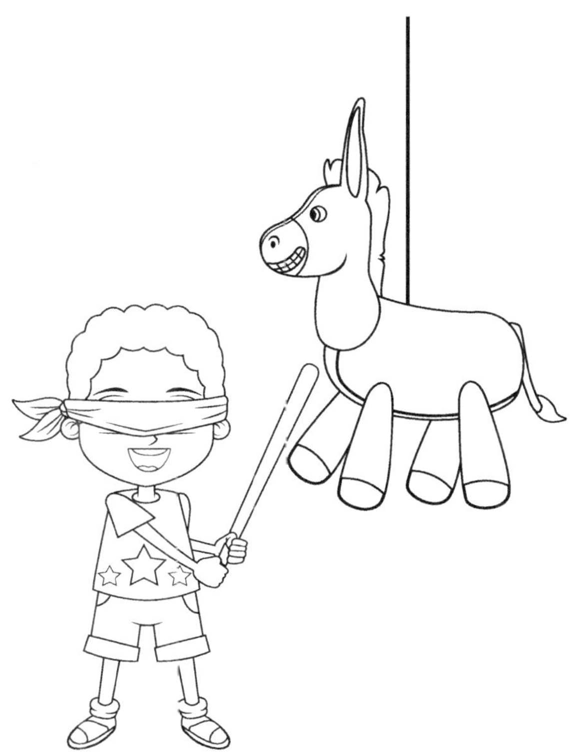

Find the Stove that is Different from the Others

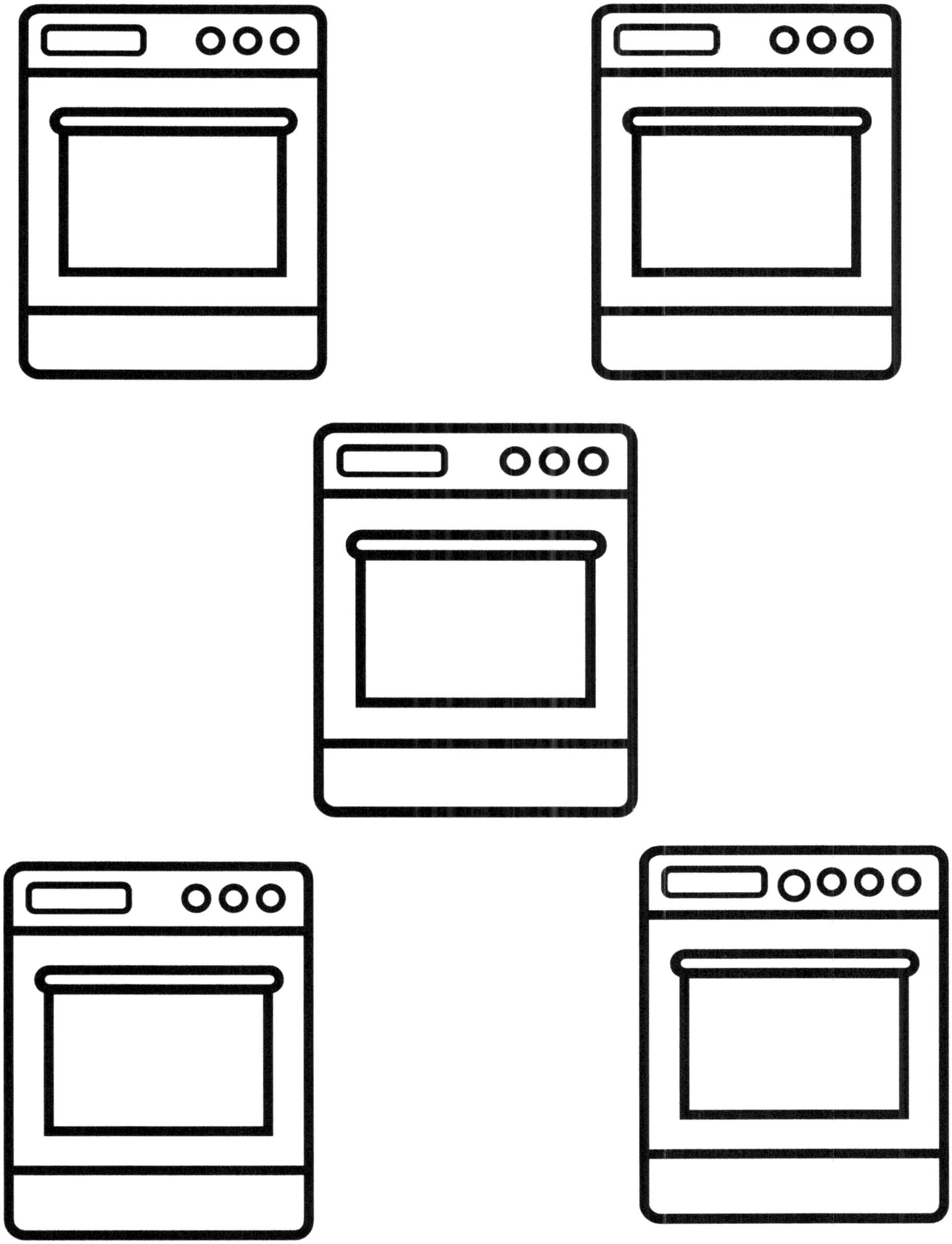

Find the Pirate Ship that is Different from the Others

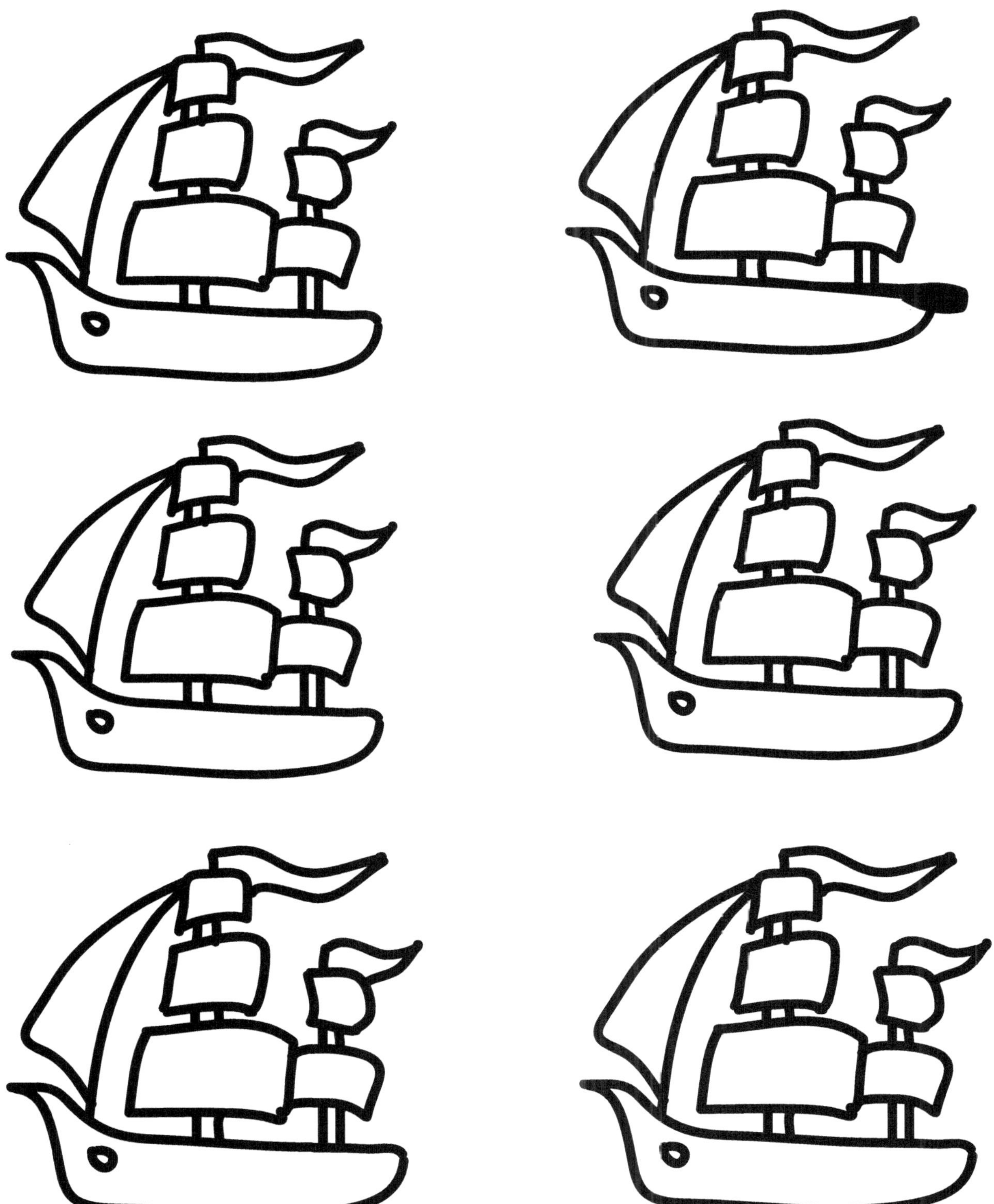

Find the Flower Pot that is Different from the Others

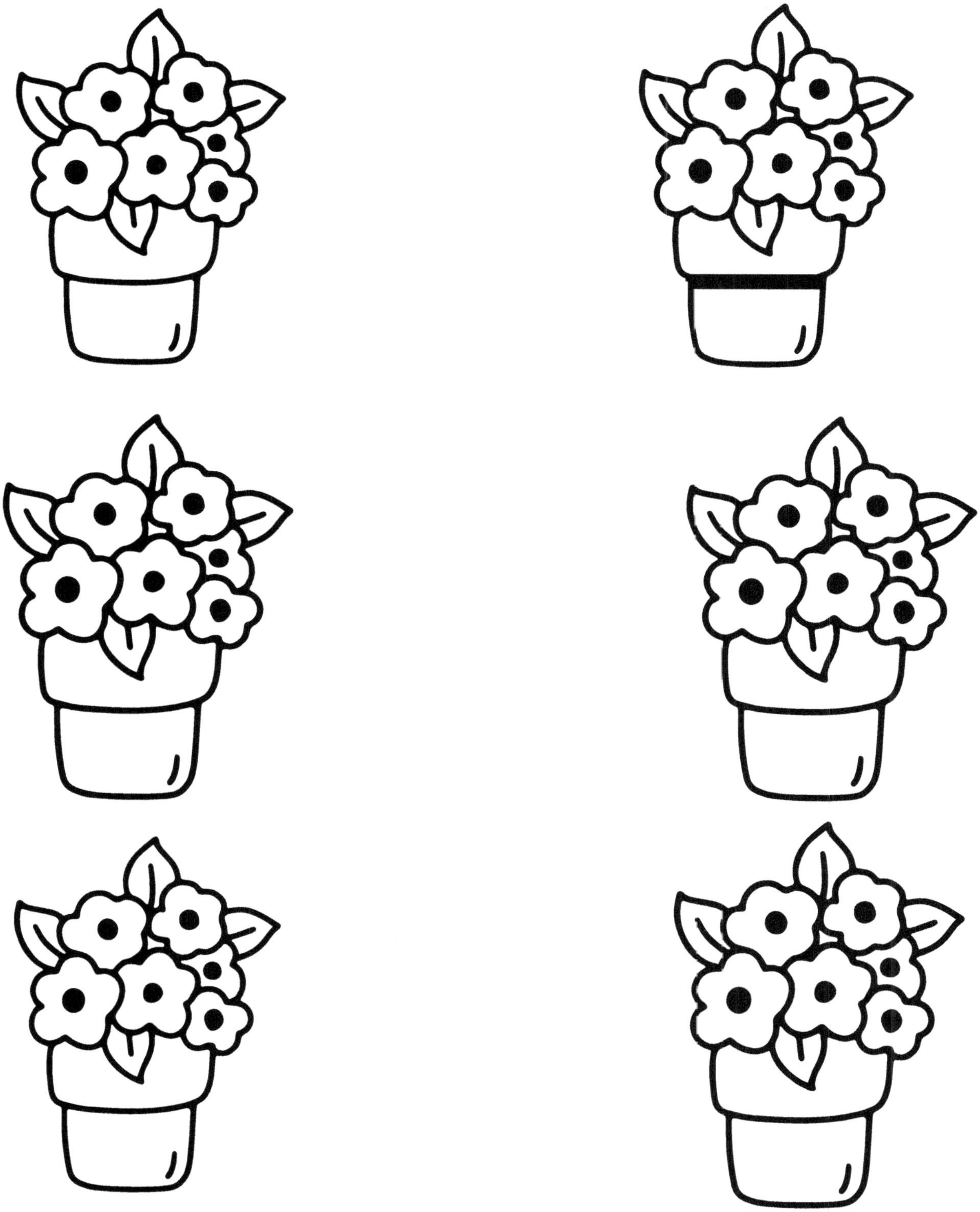

A

Circle Three Differences between the two beach pictures.

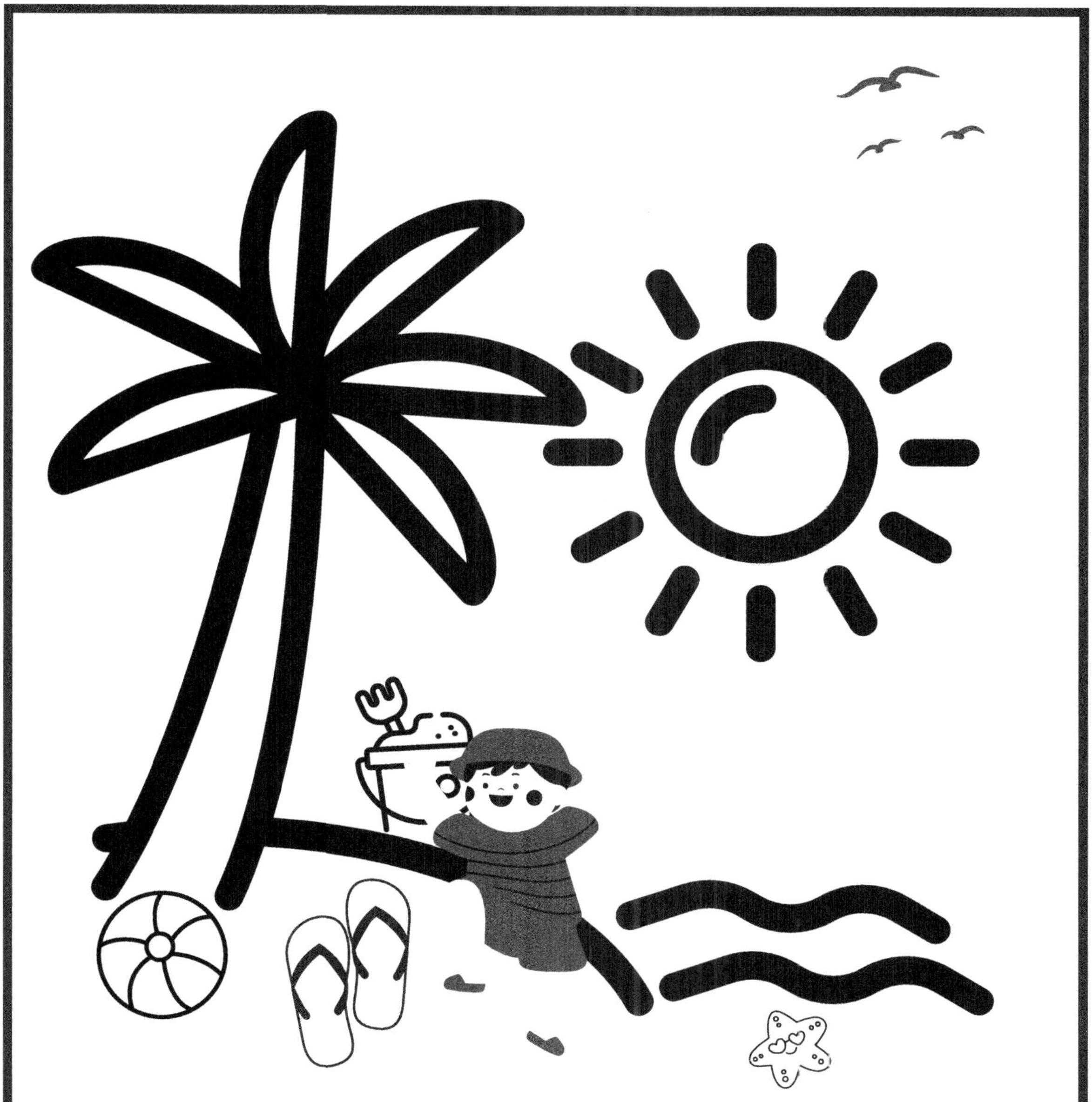

B

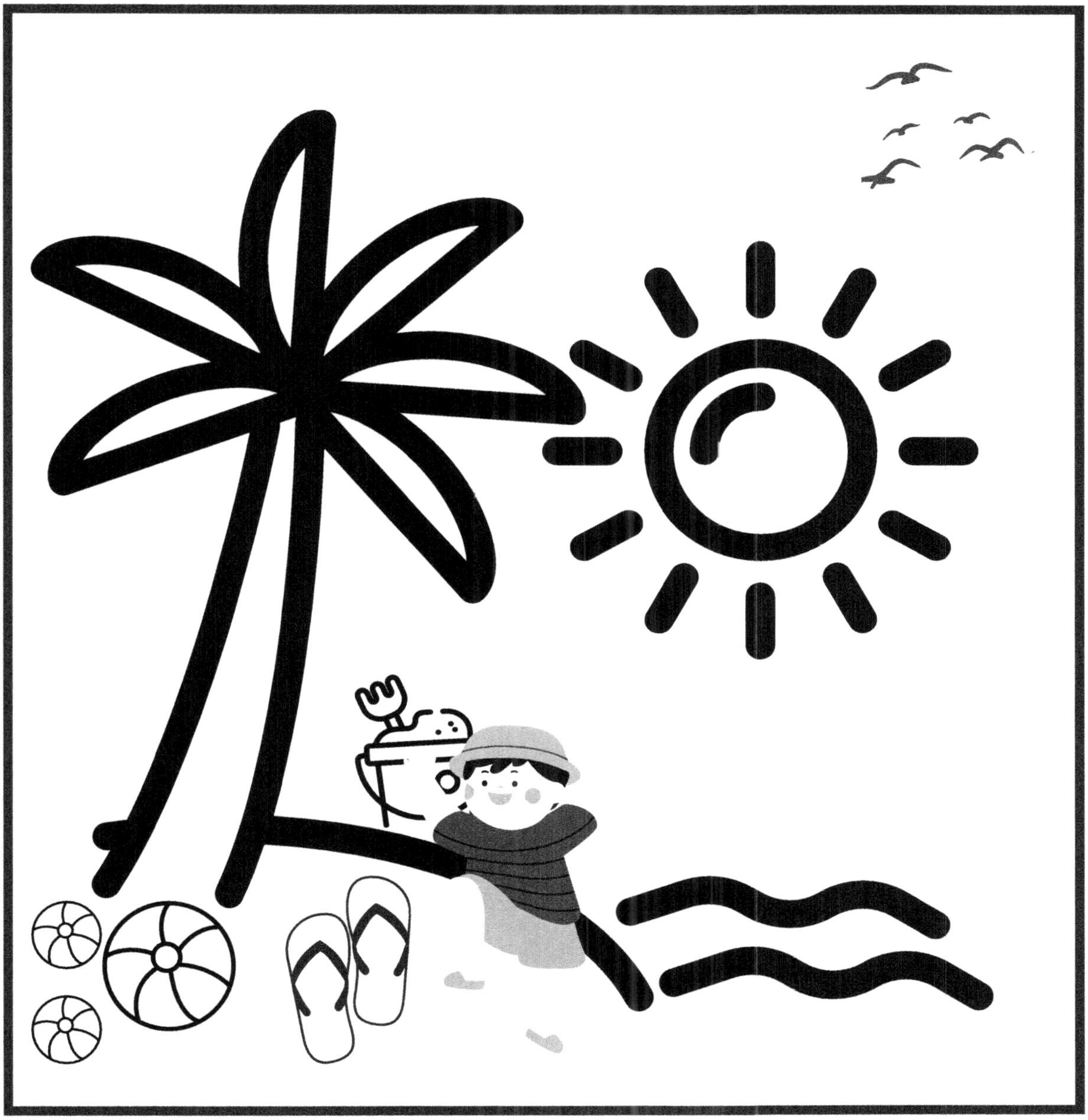

A

Circle Three Differences between the two farms.

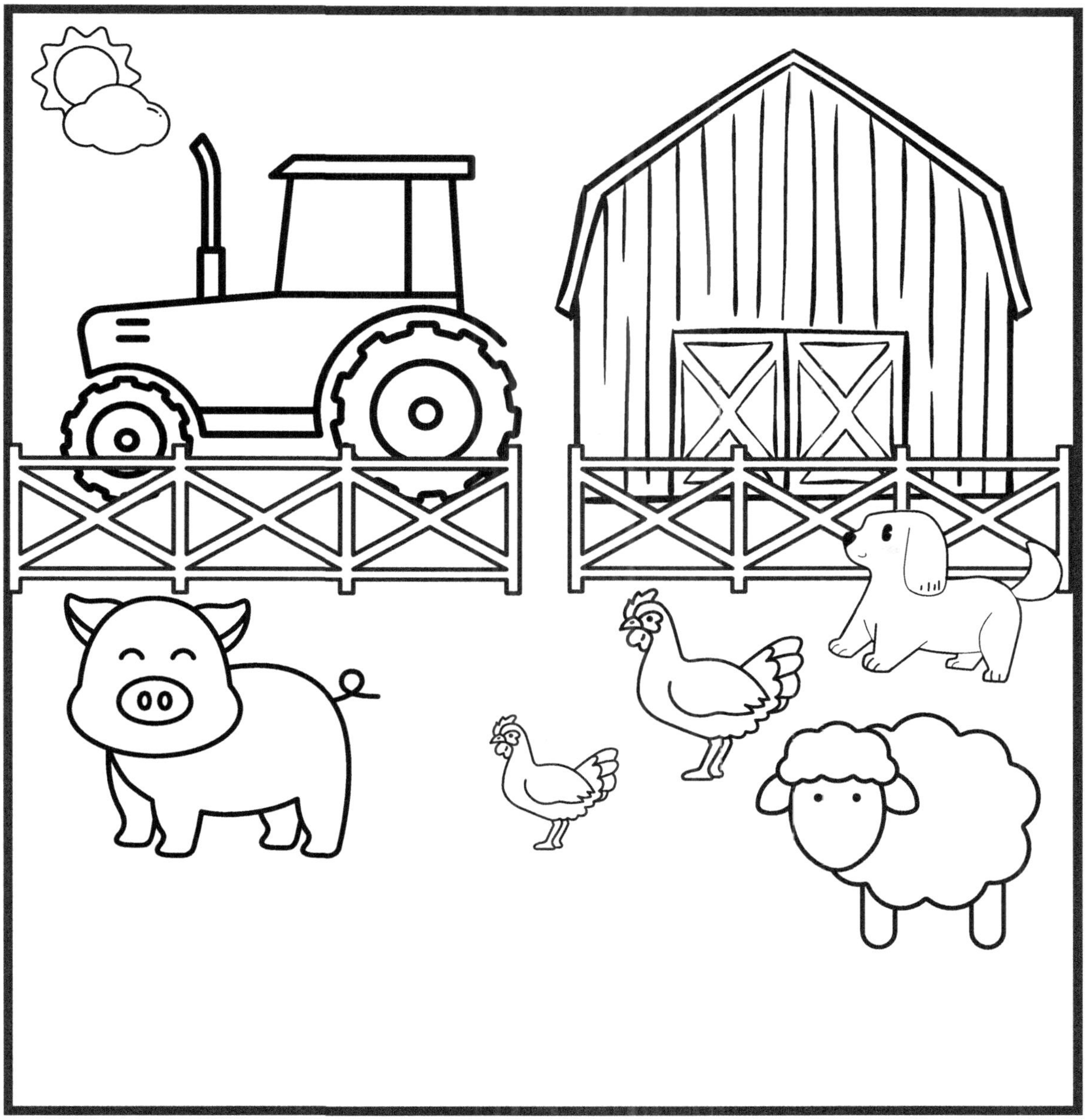

B

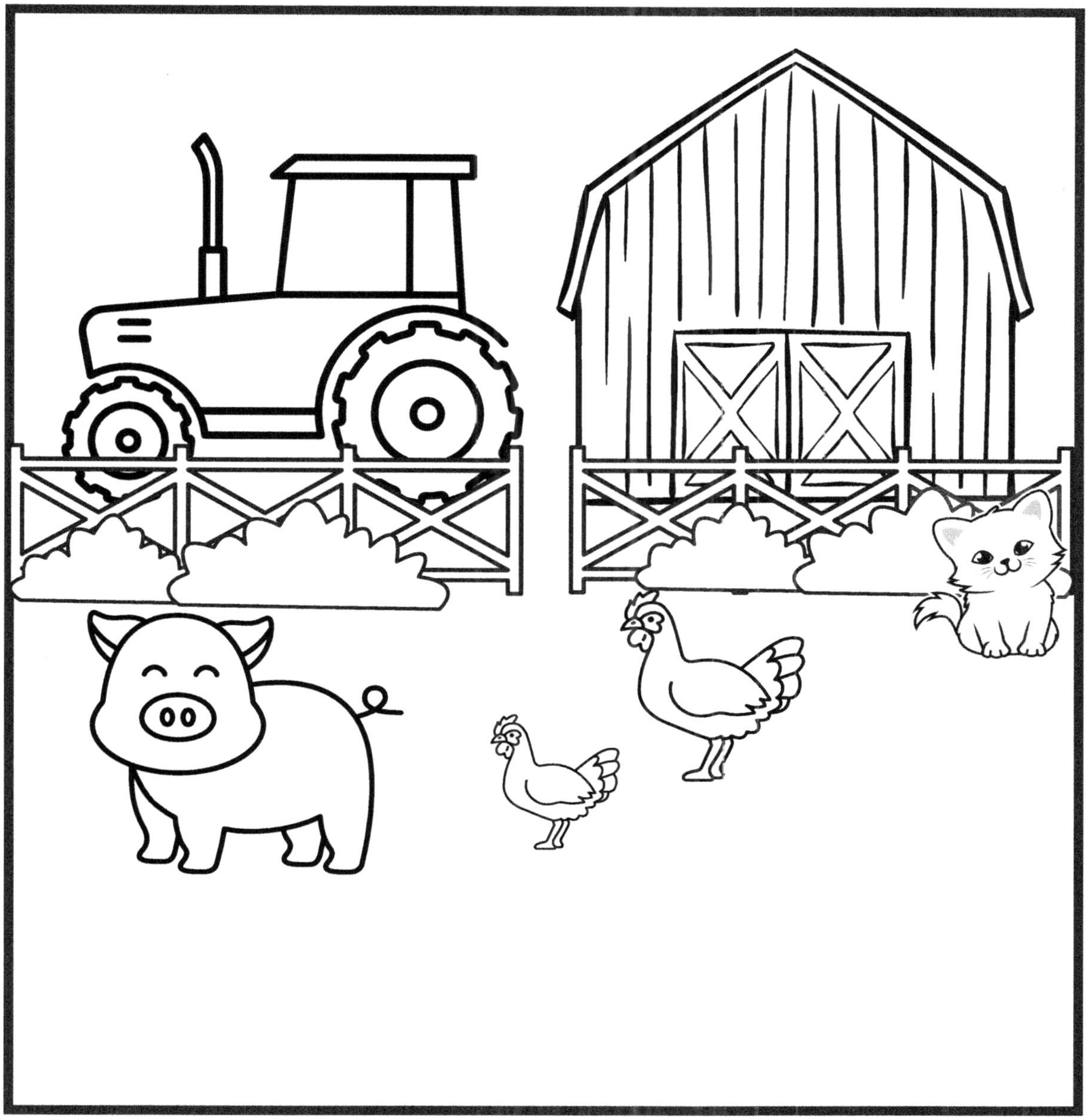

A

Circle Three Differences between the two dog parks.

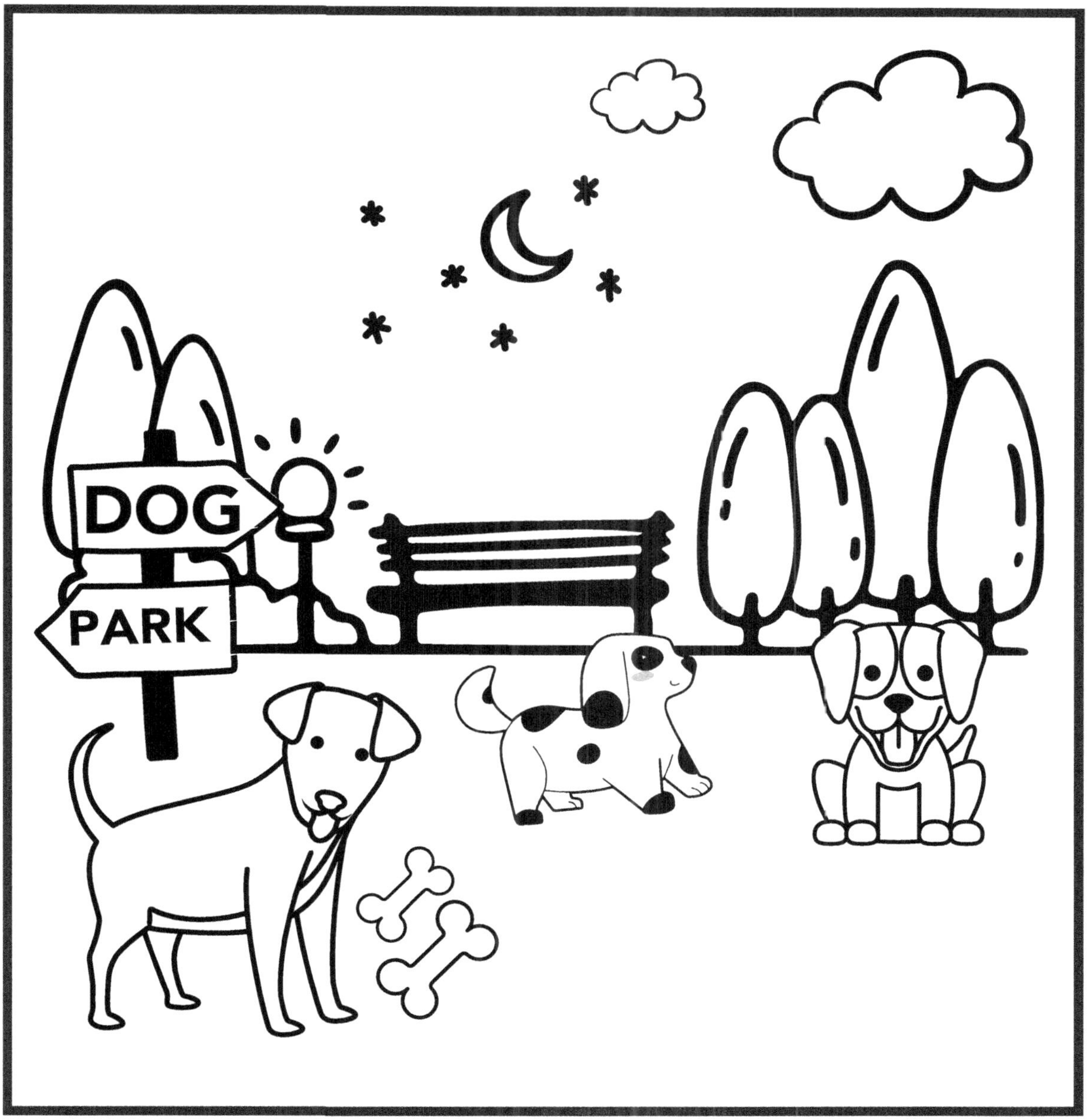

B

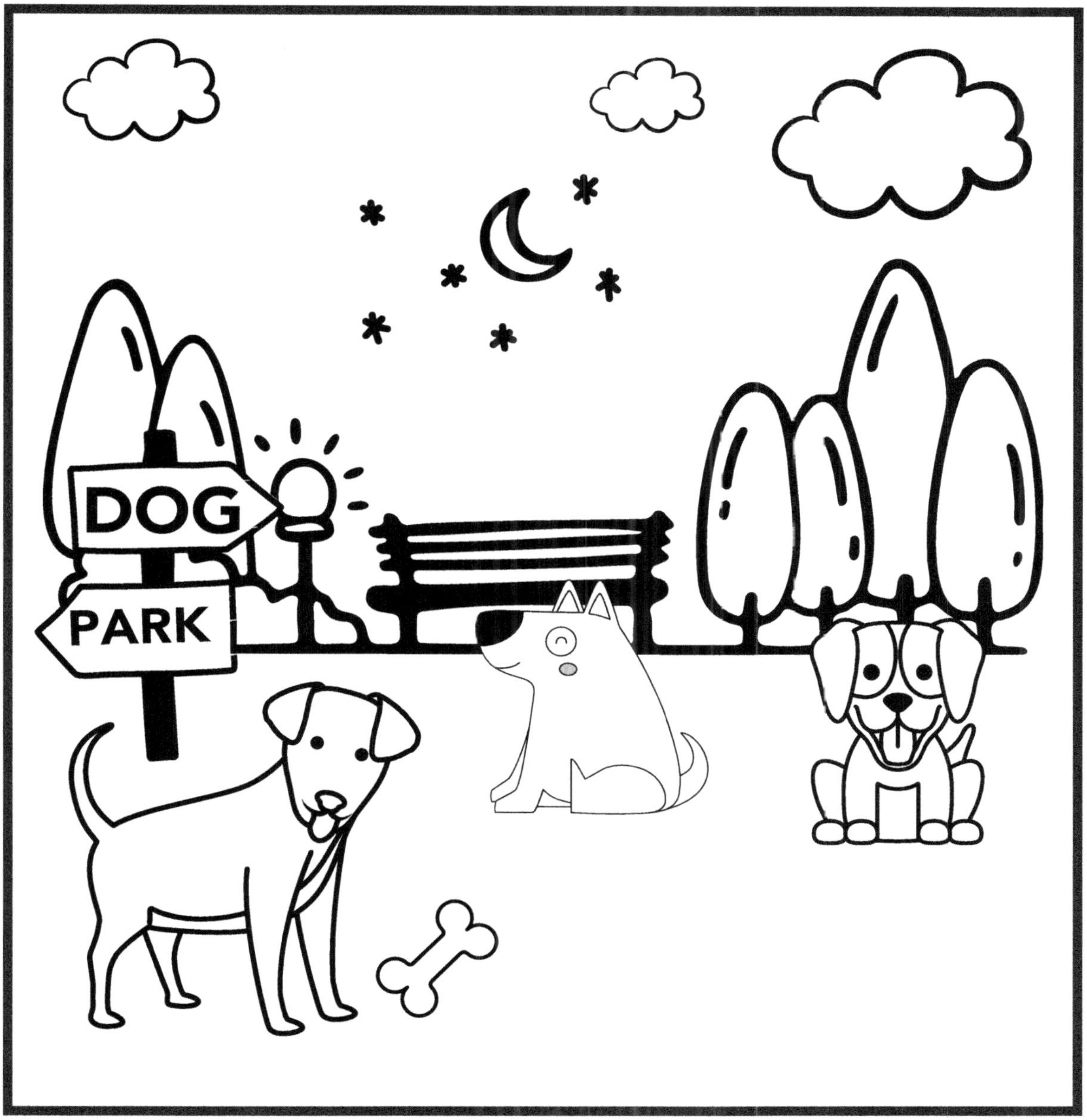

A

Circle Three Differences between the two pictures with the child riding a bicycle.

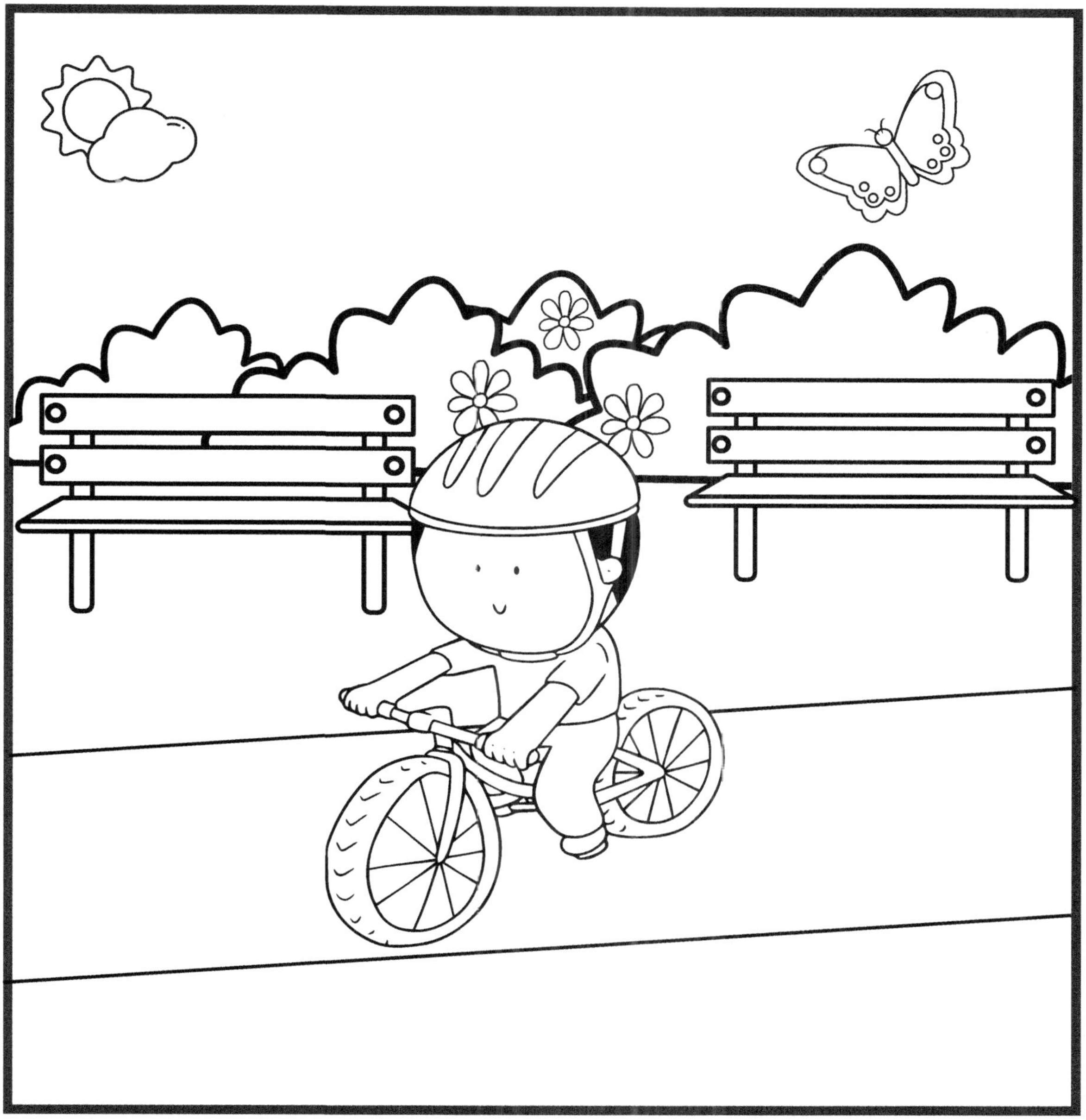

B

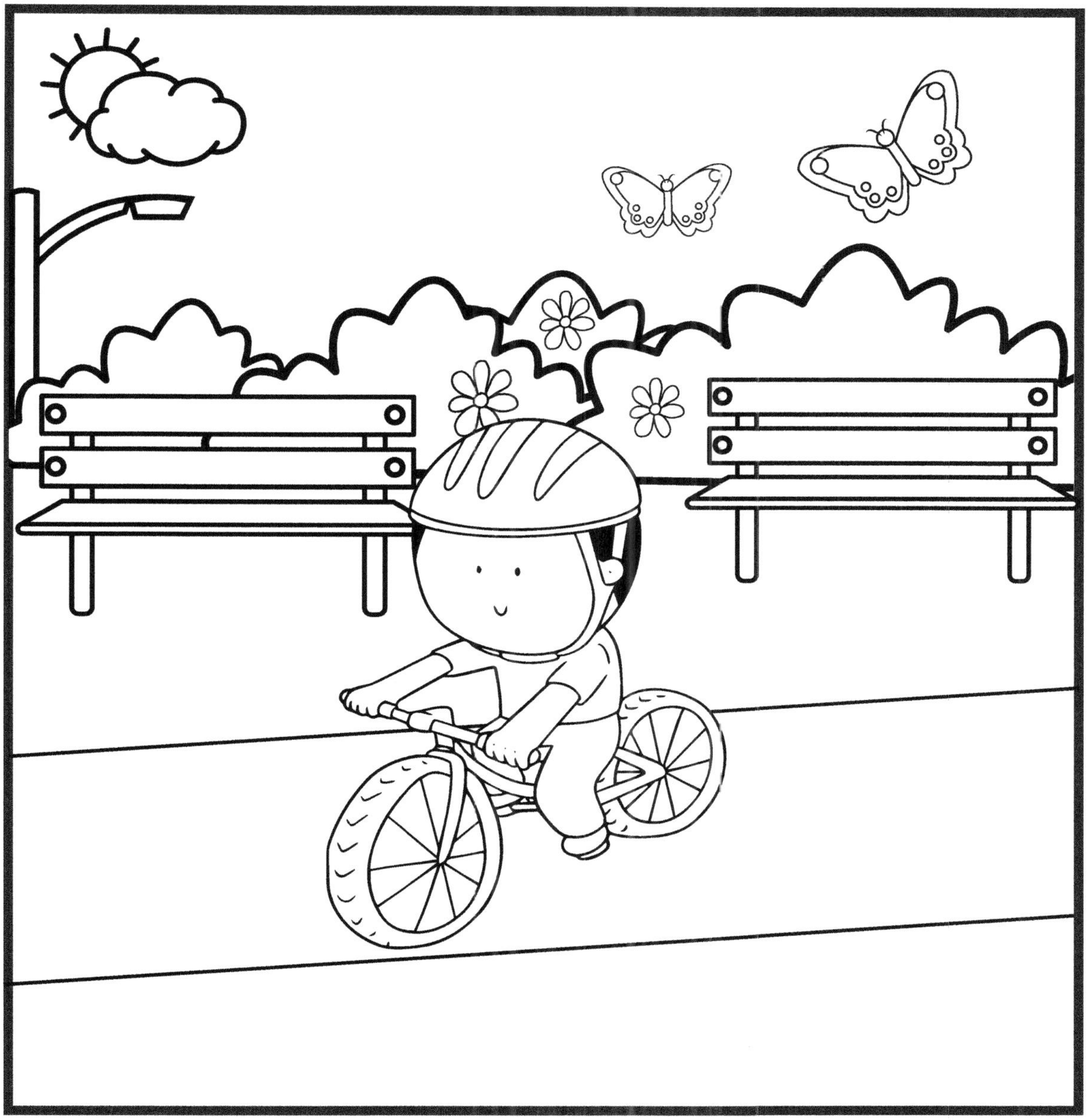

A

Circle Three Differences between the two pictures with the scuba diver.

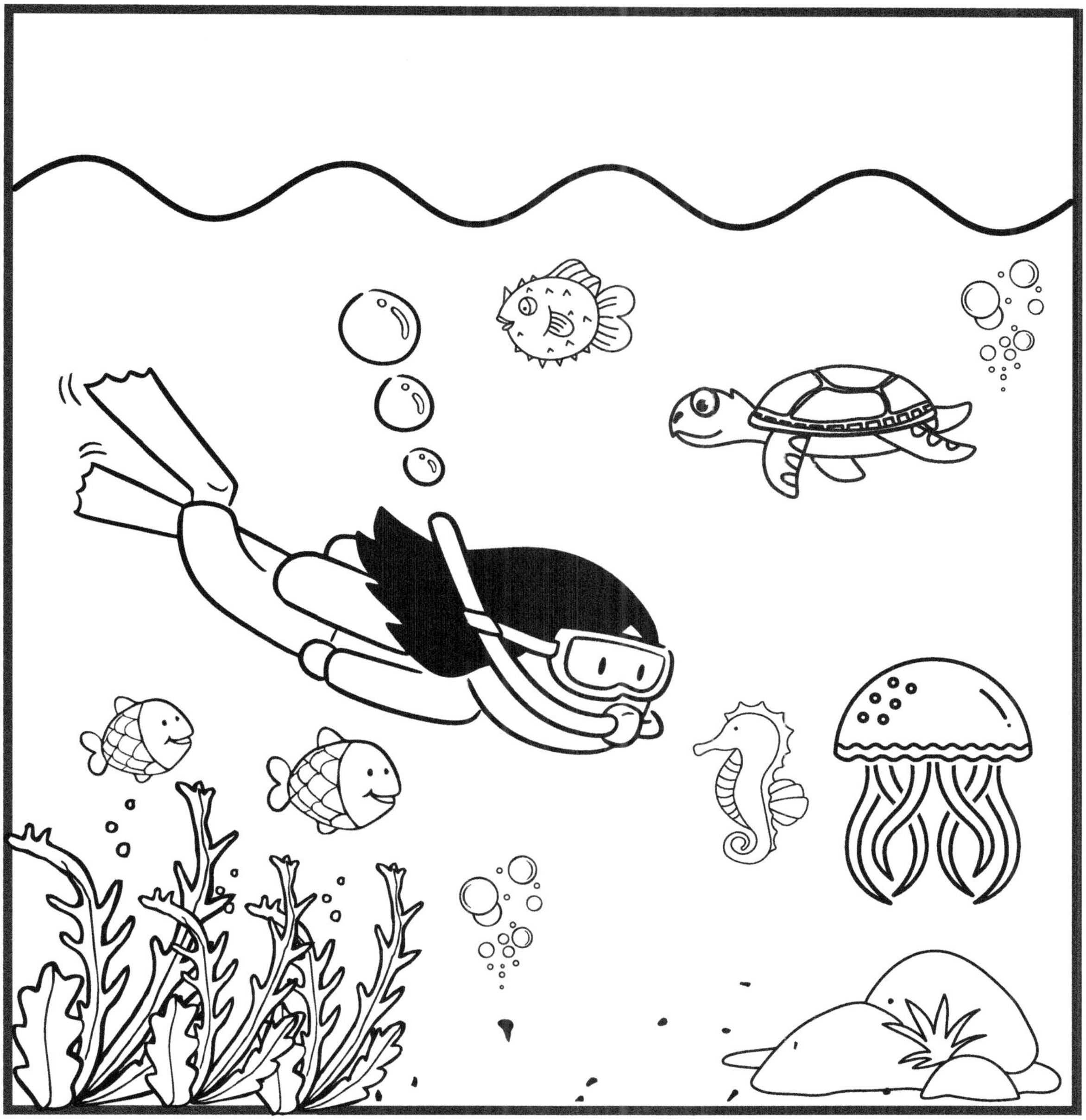

B

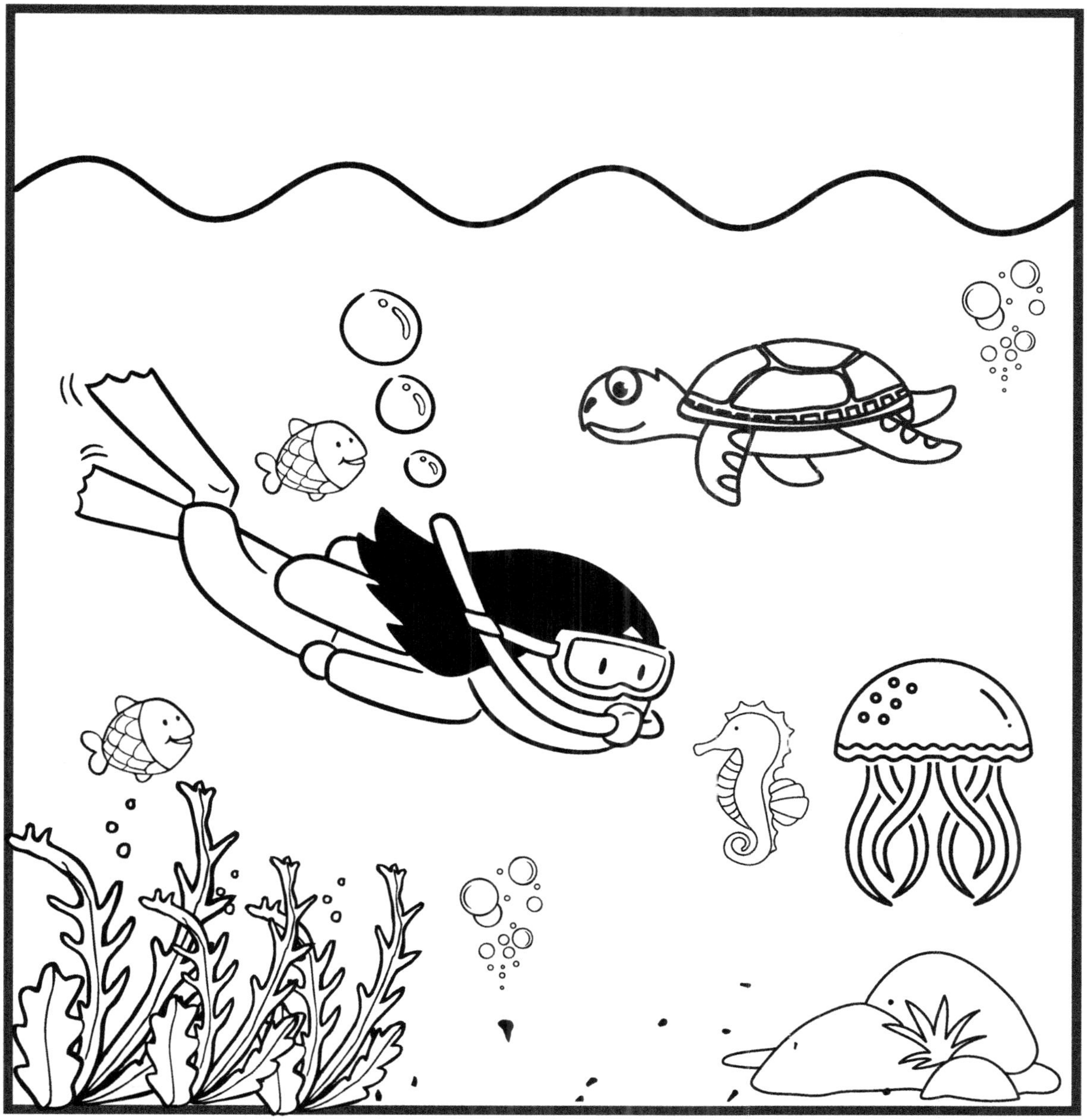

A

Circle Three Differences between the two pictures.

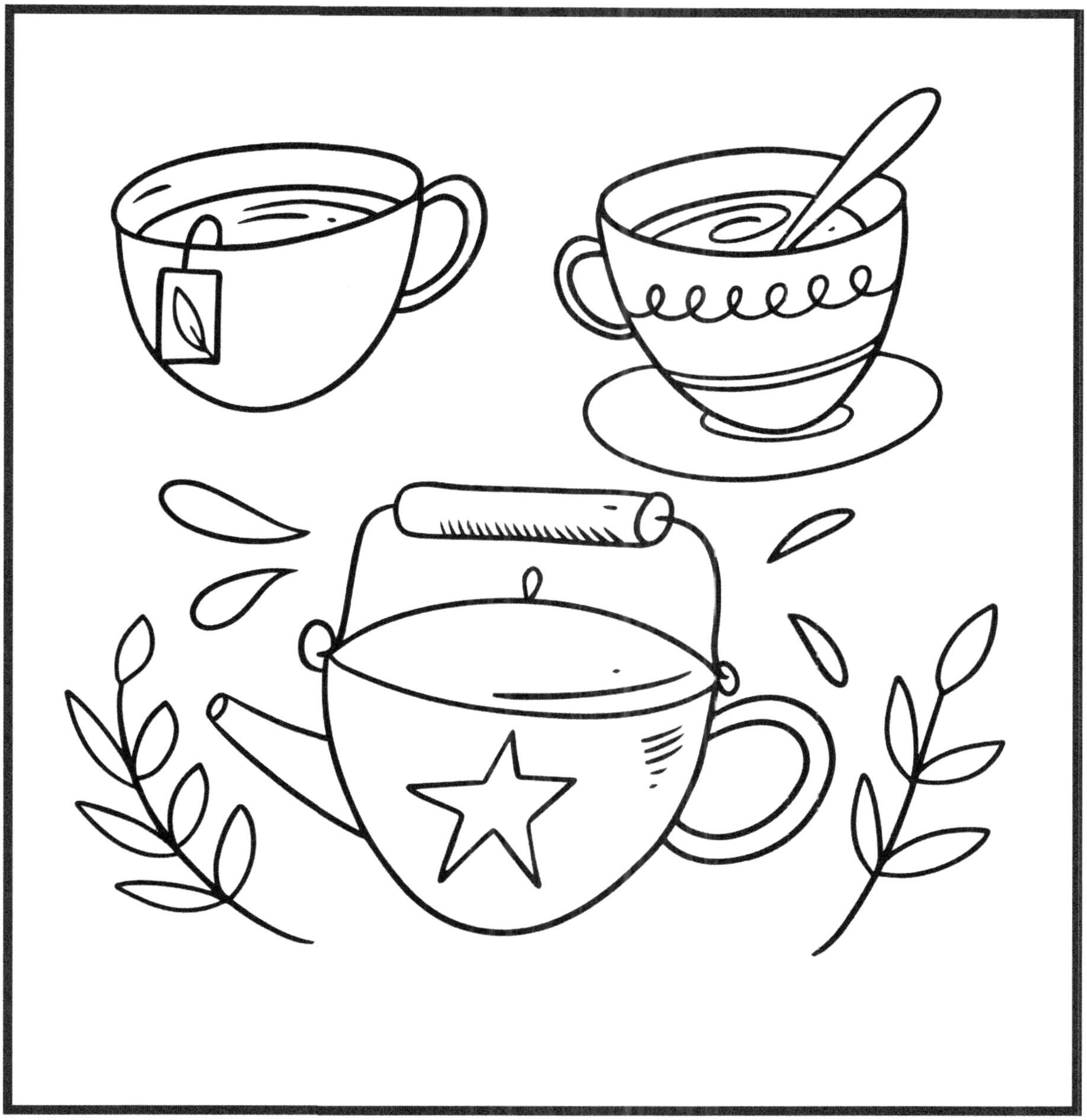

B

Circle Three Differences between the two pictures.

A

Circle Three Differences between the two Flower vases.

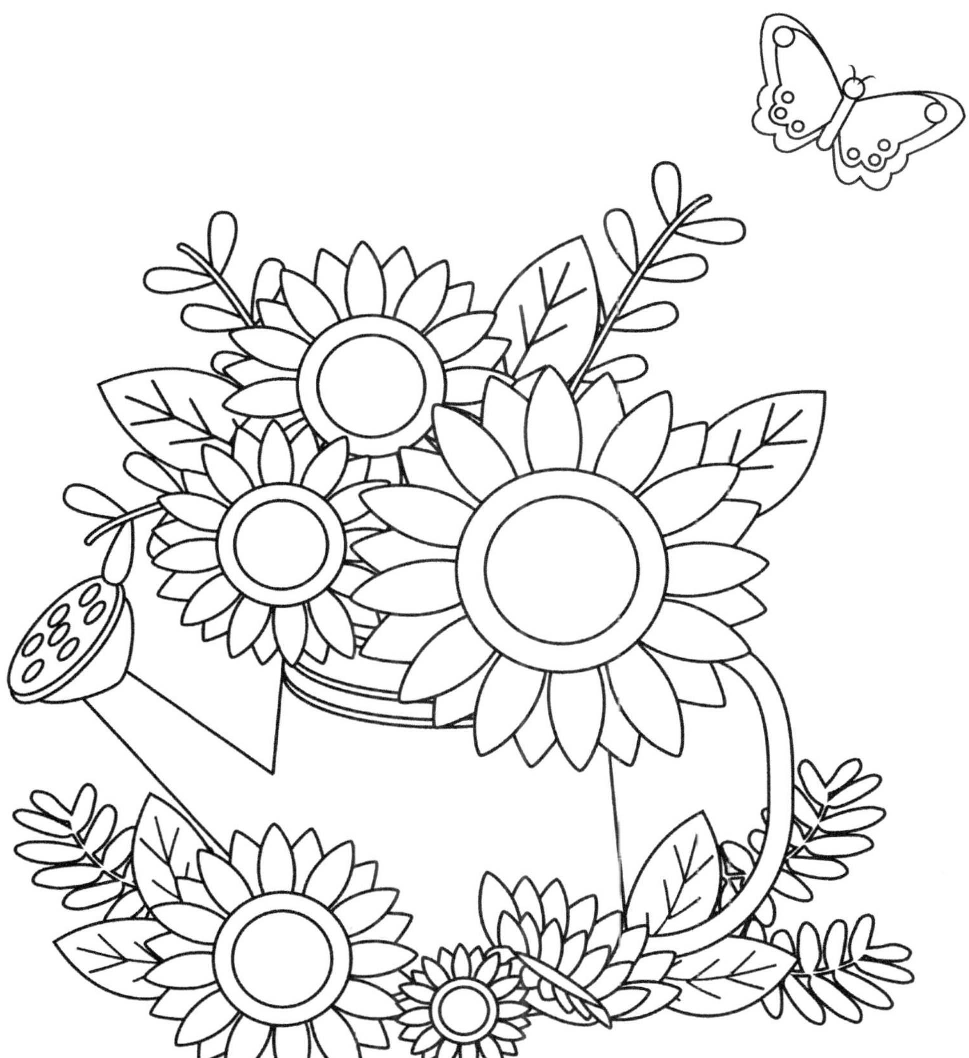

B

Circle Three Differences between the two Flower vases.

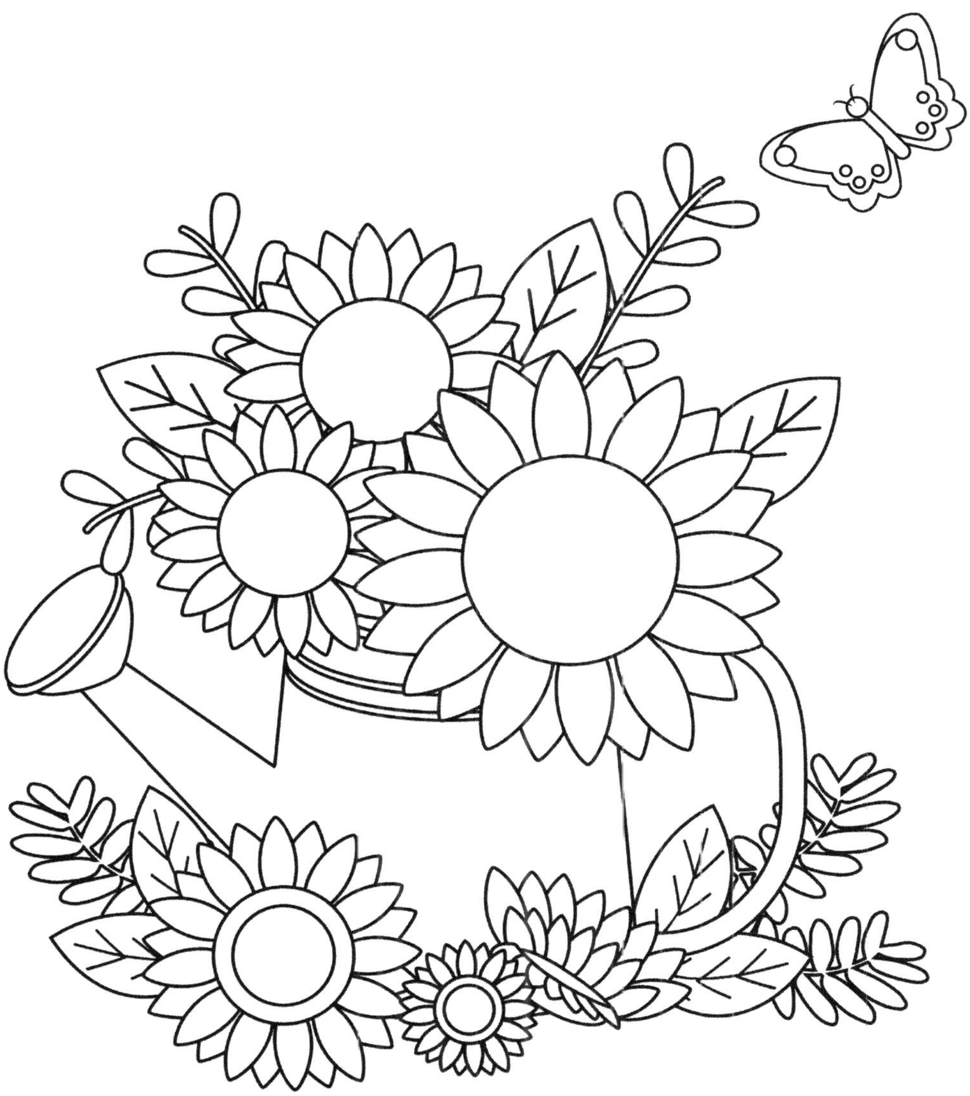

A

Circle Three Differences between the two living rooms.

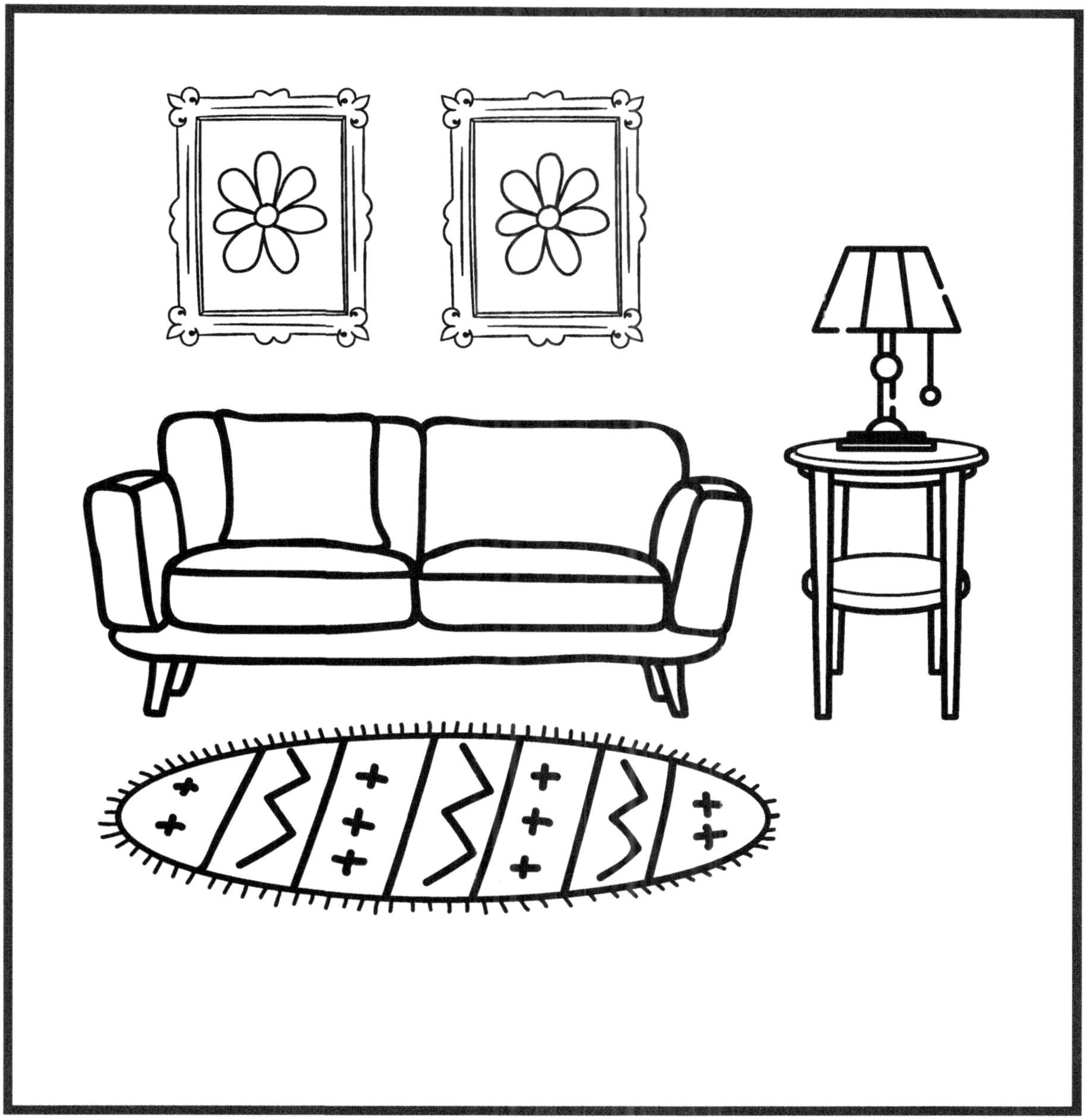

B

Circle Three Differences between the two living rooms.

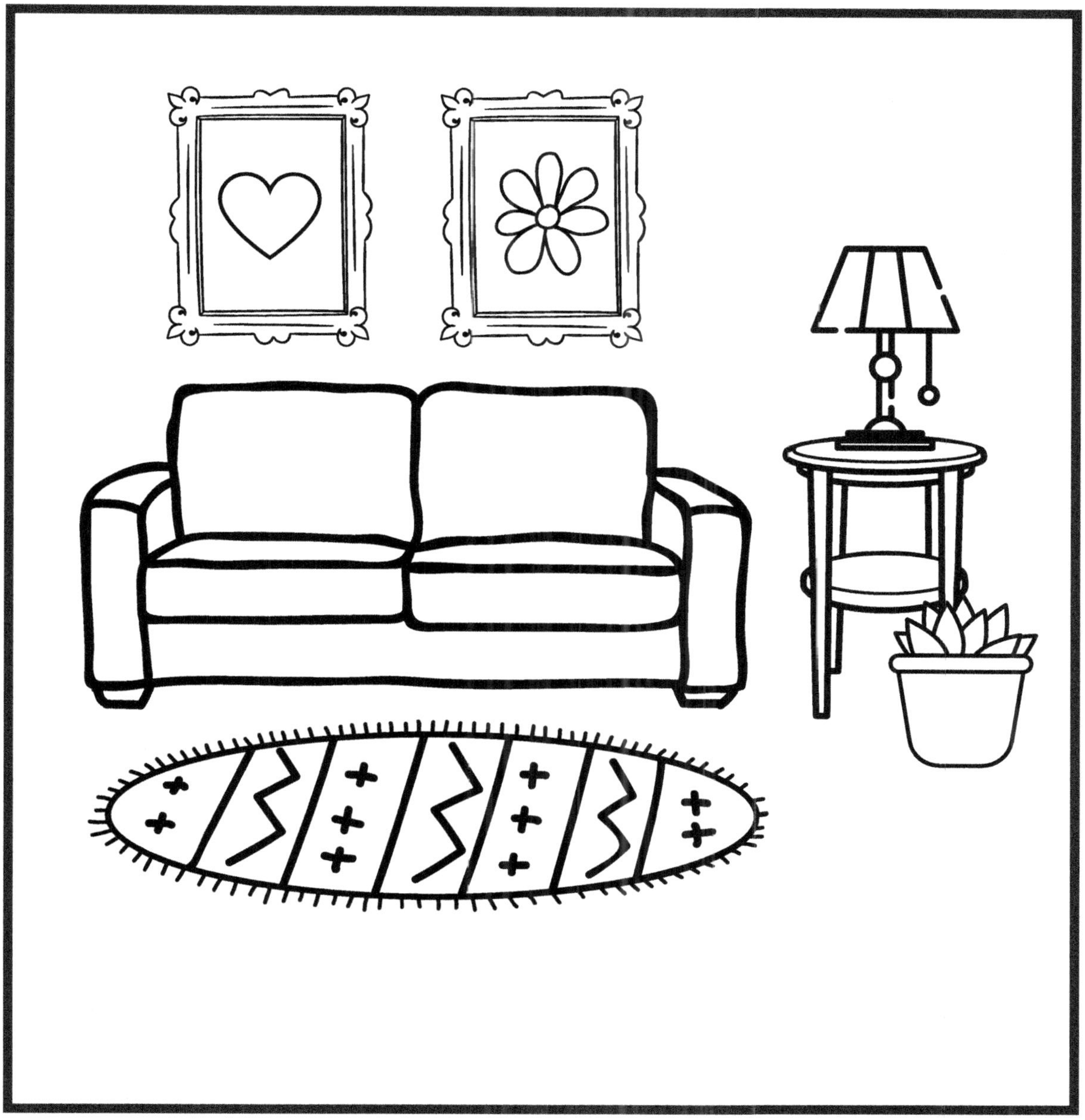

Printed in Great Britain
by Amazon

14593009R00045